Histology

AN ILLUSTRATED COLOUR TEXT

Barry S Mitchell BSc PhD MSc CSci FIBMS CBiol FIBiol
Dean, Faculty of Health and Life Sciences
De Montfort University
Leicester, UK

Sandra Peel BSc PhD DSc
Visiting Reader, Centre for Learning Anatomical Sciences
School of Medicine, University of Southampton
Southampton, UK

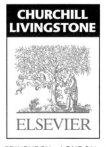
CHURCHILL
LIVINGSTONE

ELSEVIER

EDINBURGH   LONDON   NEW YORK   OXFORD   PHILADELPHIA   ST LOUIS   SYDNEY   TORONTO   2009

CHURCHILL LIVINGSTONE
ELSEVIER

First published 2009

ISBN: 9780443068539

British Library Cataloguing in Publication Data
A catalogue record for this book is available from the British Library

Library of Congress Cataloging in Publication Data
A catalog record for this book is available from the Library of Congress

ELSEVIER your source for books, journals and multimedia in the health sciences

www.elsevierhealth.com

Working together to grow libraries in developing countries

www.elsevier.com | www.bookaid.org | www.sabre.org

ELSEVIER **BOOK AID** International **Sabre Foundation**

The publisher's policy is to use paper manufactured from sustainable forests

Printed in China

Preface

Histology is more than just the science of microanatomy. It allows the examination of structures by using a variety of microscopes, but it also enables one to deduce much about the inner workings of cells, tissues and organs. It is fundamental to understanding structure and function at all levels, providing essential links between the gross dissections studied by anatomists, the functioning of the whole body studied by physiologists, and the abstract formulae representing molecules studied by biochemists. Histology therefore, underpins medical studies and many other life and applied life science studies.

This book brings together high-quality illustrations and a concise text focused on essential features. It is ideal for modern medical undergraduate curricula where basic sciences emphasise the principal points of relevance to the students. The book will also be useful for other undergraduate science courses dealing with the structure and function of animals other than humans. It will be valuable to those requiring knowledge of histology at postgraduate level (in medicine or science). It should also show the potential for using histology to advance research into the structure and function of the body.

The authors have long experience in teaching students of medicine and allied healthcare professions. This has helped to contextualise the information presented. To this end, in each chapter 'Clinical boxes' give examples of how histological changes can be indicative of ageing or disease processes. The book should help ensure that once an understanding of histology has been gained the principles of disease processes may readily be understood.

Barry Mitchell
Sandra Peel

Acknowledgements

We are particularly fortunate to have had access to histological microscope slides, most of which were produced by skilled staff of the Human Morphology Group in the School of Medicine, University of Southampton, Southampton, UK. We are extremely grateful to them for their work.

We have taken photographs of these slides especially for this book and have also used archived photographs of the slides, mostly taken by one of the authors. We are grateful to the Head of the School of Medicine, University of Southampton, Southampton, UK, for permission to use the photomicrographs. All (except one) were produced at the University of Southampton.

We thank the publishers for permission to use Fig. 6.4, which appeared in Crossman AR, Neary D. *Neuroanatomy: An Illustrated Colour Text*, 3rd edn. Elsevier: 2005.

We are grateful to Dr M. Wood for her critical reading of the manuscript.

Contents

Chapter 1
Introduction to histology

Histology is the study of the microscopic structure and function of tissues. Tissue is a general word used to describe the components of animals (and plants), and tissues consist of cells and the surrounding support media (extracellular matrix). Historically, four primary tissue types were categorised (in animals) by grouping together cells with similar form and function: they are epithelial tissue, connective tissue, muscle tissue and nerve tissue. The cells within these categories of tissues may vary in structure and be specialised according to their function and location. Most extracellular matrix is derived from the cells that it surrounds, and its composition is related to its function. For example, a very dense, hard, extracellular matrix is formed by bone cells but, in contrast, the matrix in which blood cells flow is fluid (although most blood cells do not contribute to the fluid that supports them). Various combinations of tissues form organs (e.g. the brain and liver), connecting structures (e.g. ligaments) and packing material around organs (e.g. around the kidney). In addition, various combinations of organs and other structures form systems of the body which together perform related functions (see Chapters 10–16).

The unaided (good) eye can just about see objects which are 200 μm in diameter; very few cells are as big as this, although a very fine hair may be this width. However, there are particular challenges in examining structures smaller than 200 μm. Most components of tissues have little colour and contrast, and thus cells and the matrices surrounding them are indistinguishable if light is transmitted through them using a basic light microscope. Indeed, light will only penetrate thin slices of tissues or thin layers of cells growing in vitro. Various types of microscopes and methods of preparing specimens for examination have been developed. Living, isolated, whole cells can be examined using special (phase contrast) light microscopes but contrast is limited and the cells rarely have around them the structures they had in the body. In routine histology, very thin slices of tissues (5–10 μm thick) are prepared through which light can penetrate. To achieve sufficient contrast and colours in the tissues so that they may be visualised, dyes or specific chemicals are applied to the slices of tissues. In these specimens, light microscopy can resolve detail of structures about 0.2 μm apart. However, by using much thinner slices and electrons instead of light, electron microscopy can resolve detail down to about 0.0002 μm. (Note 1 mm = 1000 μm.)

Numerous advanced techniques, suitable for light and electron microscopy, may be used to identify specific molecules in tissues via their reaction with labelled molecules. The labelled molecule is then detected, e.g. as colour using ordinary light microscopy, as fluorescence by viewing using ultraviolet light or as radioactivity using photographic film. Details of advanced techniques for studying the components of tissues with light and electron microscopes are beyond the scope of this book and the reader is advised to consult other texts. However, we give a brief overview below of basic histological techniques.

Tissue preservation (fixation)

If any piece of the living body is removed it begins to degenerate as cell death occurs: this process is referred to as necrosis. In this process, enzymes in cells are released from their normal location and break down the cells and molecules in surrounding areas. Consequently, the precise three-dimensional arrangement of structures within, and surrounding, cells in life disappears. To study the arrangement of molecules, cells, extracellular matrix, tissues and organs as they were in life, necrosis must be prevented and the molecules, cells, etc. must be preserved. There are various methods for preservation, but a standard way is to place samples of tissue in a solution of formaldehyde as rapidly as possible after death or after removing them from a living body. Formaldehyde changes the conformational state of the proteins (and other large molecules) and prevents enzymes from degrading the tissues: this process is known as fixation. This chemical fixation can be compared with the process of boiling an egg in which heat changes the conformational state of the proteins and, with enough boiling, the proteins in the white and yolk of the egg become solid.

Tissue processing for slicing (sectioning)

Most body tissues are soft in life and only a little harder after they have been fixed in formaldehyde, so they are difficult to slice thinly enough to be examined using a routine microscope. In order to prepare thin slices, tissue samples are impregnated with a substance which makes them solid. The medium used in routine histology to confer rigidity is paraffin wax, which is liquid at about 58°C but solid at room temperature. Wax and water-based tissues are immiscible, so formaldehyde-fixed tissue samples cannot be impregnated directly with wax. Hence, tissue samples are processed through a schedule which removes and replaces the water. This is most easily achieved by transferring the tissue sample through gradually increasing concentrations of alcohol which (at 100%) replaces all the water. Alcohol itself is also immiscible with wax but it is replaced in the tissue sample by processing it through increasing concentrations of a solvent that is miscible with alcohol and wax, e.g. chloroform or xylene. This solvent in turn is removed by placing the tissue sample in several changes of molten wax so that the wax infiltrates the tissue.

The sample in the molten wax is then allowed to set and a solid block of wax forms in which the tissue sample is embedded. The tissue is then ready for sectioning. Given the toxicity of the substances used in these processes, appropriate safety precautions must be taken.

Advanced techniques make use of a variety of solid support media, e.g. a hard synthetic resin may be used to embed tissue samples and very thin sections (0.1 μm) cut and examined using an electron microscope. In addition, by freezing a tissue sample immediately after removing it from a living body an instant support medium of ice is formed. Sectioning can be done at sub-zero temperature and provide histological preparations which can be examined within minutes of sampling. This is a routine process that is of use to surgeons in deciding how to proceed with an operation.

Tissue sectioning

Thin sections (slices) are cut using a microtome, a machine that holds an embedded tissue sample firmly in place and cuts thin sections with a very sharp blade. Typically, a wax-embedded tissue sample can be cut at 5 μm thick. The sections are then placed on glass microscope slides ready for staining procedures to allow visualisation of the components of the tissue sample.

Methods for visualising tissues for light microscopy

As most staining methods use dyes soluble in water, wax-embedded tissue sections have to be processed through the reverse of the sequence of solvents used to embed the tissues in order to remove the wax and return the tissue sample to an aqueous solution.

Many staining methods depend on the chemical attraction of dyes for particular molecular configurations in tissues. The most common technique used to demonstrate the general topography of tissues uses the dyes haematoxylin and eosin (H&E). About half the illustrations in this book are of photomicrographs of sections stained with the H&E method. Other illustrations are of sections prepared using special methods as indicated in the text and captions.

H&E method

Haematoxylin is a basic dye which binds to acidic components in tissues, producing a blue/purple colour. Typically, haematoxylin binds to nuclei because of their content of deoxyribonucleic acid (DNA) and ribonucleic acid (RNA). Nuclei containing mostly inactive DNA appear as densely stained structures in H&E-stained sections (Fig. 1.1). In some instances, parts of the nuclei appear palely stained, and this indicates that the DNA is uncoiled and was in active use prior to fixation. In addition, in some palely stained nuclei a small, dense, round region of staining may be apparent; this is a nucleolus (Fig. 1.1). The dense staining, by haematoxylin, of the RNA in a nucleolus indicates that the cell was actively synthesising protein (see Chapter 2). Cells synthesising large amounts of protein also contain large amounts of RNA in their cytoplasm, and this too may be visualised as it will bind haematoxylin and appear bluish purple (Fig. 1.1). In contrast, eosin is an acidic dye and binds to bases. The proteins in the cytoplasm of many cells (Fig. 1.1) and proteins in extracellular matrices stain with eosin and appear red or pinkish orange.

Histochemistry and immunohistochemistry

In contrast to staining with dyes, histochemistry and immunohistochemistry techniques involve specific chemical or immunological reactions to detect various components of tissues. For example, histochemistry can be used to detect types, and location, of carbohydrates (Fig. 1.2) and enzymes. Immunohistochemistry can detect molecules that are antigens by applying labelled antibodies that can be visualised using a microscope. It is beyond the scope of this book to detail the range of methods available for demonstrating specific molecules in tissues.

Illustrations in this book

Most illustrations in this book were photographed on a Zeiss or an Olympus light microscope using lenses which magnify between ×12 and ×120. (Some blood cells were photographed using lenses magnifying at about ×350.) Some images were photographed using colour-positive transparency film (about 10 × 13 cm), others using 35 mm film (negative and positive) and others using a digital camera with optical magnification of ×4 in addition to magnification by microscope lenses. Over half of the illustrations using light microscopy were taken especially for this book. The other images using light and electron microscopy are from material prepared and archived by the Human Morphology Group at the University of Southampton, Southampton, UK, and are

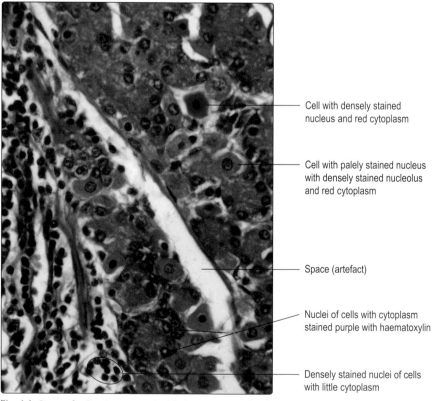

Cell with densely stained nucleus and red cytoplasm

Cell with palely stained nucleus with densely stained nucleolus and red cytoplasm

Space (artefact)

Nuclei of cells with cytoplasm stained purple with haematoxylin

Densely stained nuclei of cells with little cytoplasm

Fig. 1.1 **Stomach.** Routine wax-embedded section stained with haematoxylin and eosin. Medium magnification.

currently in the Centre for Learning Anatomical Sciences, School of Medicine, University of Southampton.

Interpretation in histology

One of the challenges in interpreting structure and function by studying histological sections is how to assess the size of objects viewed (when using a microscope or viewing an illustration). If red blood cells can be identified, they can be used as a rough scale to estimate the size of other structures as their maximum diameter is about 7 μm (Fig. 1.3). Not all red cells will be sectioned

through their largest diameter, so care needs to be taken when assessing the size of other structures in comparison with red cells.

Another challenge in interpreting sections of tissues is that a variety of appearances may result from slicing three-dimensional structures and examining them as very thin slices, effectively as two-dimensional structures. Consider slicing a curved, peeled banana (Fig. 1.4). Taking a slice along its length will show the curve and that it is a solid object. Slicing at right angles to the length of a banana will produce circular (solid) slices which will be smaller in diameter

if sliced close to an end rather than in the middle. Obliquely cut slices will produce solid ellipsoid shapes which will vary in shape and size depending on the angle of cut. Histological sections on microscope slides have to be interpreted by constructing possible three-dimensional shapes from their two-dimensional appearance. For example, if a hollow circular structure is seen in a histological section it may be from a hollow sphere or part of a straight or coiled hollow tube cut at right angles to its length.

Artefacts present other challenges in interpreting histological sections. Artefacts are appearances in histological sections which are there as a consequence of procedures used to prepare the tissue sample. During fixation, e.g. with formaldehyde, many small water-soluble molecules are not 'fixed' in place, and even those molecules that are fixed in place may shrink and pull away from adjacent structures. Spaces seen in histological sections (Figs 1.1–1.3) have to be assessed and their cause (artefact or not) determined. Experience and knowledge of the structures being examined helps to identify the space in Fig. 1.1 as an artefact. In contrast, the space in Fig. 1.2 is not an artefact: it is part of the empty lumen of the small intestine. Other empty spaces in tissue samples may be due to the extraction of fat by the organic solvents used in routine histological processing or to components not reacting with the stains used. The apparently large, empty spaces in Fig. 1.3 show the typical appearance of adipose cells. These are cells in which

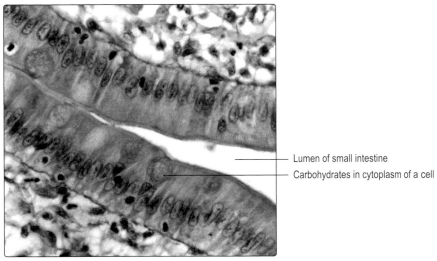

Lumen of small intestine
Carbohydrates in cytoplasm of a cell

Fig. 1.2 **Small intestine.** Routine wax-embedded section stained with special stain which displays certain large carbohydrate molecules as blue/turquoise. High magnification.

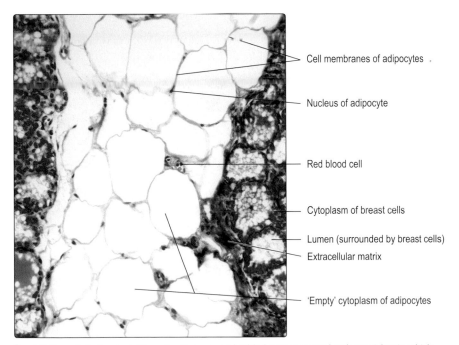

Cell membranes of adipocytes
Nucleus of adipocyte
Red blood cell
Cytoplasm of breast cells
Lumen (surrounded by breast cells)
Extracellular matrix
'Empty' cytoplasm of adipocytes

Fig. 1.3 **Breast during lactation.** Routine wax-embedded section stained with special stain which shows extracellular proteins as blue. Red cells appear scarlet. Compare the size of the red cells with the size of the adipose cells. (Adipose cells are some of the largest cells in the body and red cells are about 7 μm in diameter.) Low magnification.

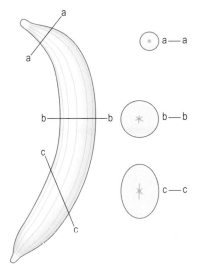

Fig. 1.4 **A banana showing the appearance of slices taken across various planes.**
Sections a–a and b–b are transverse sections and section c–c is an oblique section.

fat occupies most of the cytoplasm. Routine processing extracted the fat and only the nucleus and membrane around each adipose cell is seen. In Fig. 1.2, the cells which have been stained blue due to their carbohydrate content would have bound little or no H&E and would thus have appeared empty in a routine preparation.

Another challenge presented, especially to histopathologists and researchers, is to decide whether the tissue section examined is normal or abnormal. In some instances, if the tissue has not been fixed rapidly after death, necrosis occurs and this changes the appearance of the sectioned tissue. In addition, histopathologists and researchers have to be able to interpret the appearance of a tissue sample and consider the tissue in relation to time in the context of the whole body. Interpreting what has gone before may allow a diagnosis of a disease. Predicting what might yet happen to a patient could be essential, especially if the tissue sample shows signs of cancer. Consider looking at a sliced hard boiled egg (described above as an example of fixation). Consider the two-dimensional slice of the egg in the context of time. What would it have been like 20 or so days earlier before boiling (fixation), or what might it have become 20 days later if it had not been boiled?

Summary

- Histology is the study of the microscopic structure and function of tissues.
- Components of the body are categorised as four tissue types: epithelial, connective, muscle and nerve. Tissues comprise cells and extracellular material which carry out specific functions.
- Various combinations of tissues form organs and other components of the body.

In order to examine the microscopic structure of tissues, various procedures are necessary. The routine processes for doing this are:

- *Fixation*. Tissues are immersed in formaldehyde, which preserves the molecules and their structural arrangement in tissues as near as possible to how they were in life (and prevents necrosis).
- *Processing*. These stages replace the water with solvents that are miscible with molten wax.
- *Embedding*. Tissues in molten wax are cooled and the solid wax supports the tissue.
- *Sectioning*. Thin slices of wax-embedded tissue are cut and attached to microscope slides.
- *Processing*. This removes the wax and returns the tissues to an aqueous state.
- *Staining*. This allows tissue components to be visualised. Haematoxylin stains acidic substances (e.g. DNA in nuclei) blue/purple and eosin stains basic substances (e.g. many cytoplasmic proteins) red/orange.

Interpretation of microscopic structure may involve assessing:

- possible three-dimensional structures represented by a two-dimensional image
- the size and identity of structures (including their chemical composition) and their function
- whether any appearance is due to artefacts
- the significance of time in respect of the tissue sample, e.g. does it show that if similar tissue remains in the body it could be harmful.

Chapter 2
The cell

Cells are the fundamental units of life. Textbooks may describe a 'typical' cell, but such a cell does not exist. Most cells are, to some extent, specialised in terms of their structure and function. Accordingly, the structural appearance of cells can provide information about their function. The term used to describe how cells are specialised is 'differentiation'. Most cells have a nucleus which contains molecular programmes encoded in DNA (in chromosomes) that direct how a cell differentiates and what function(s) it performs. Many types of cell, even some which are differentiated, also have the ability to replicate themselves by a process of cell division known as mitosis (see below). Mitotic activity may continue in many types of cell throughout the life of the individual. Cells undergoing successive rounds of mitosis are described as passing through a series of events known as the cell cycle (see below). Other cells may reach an end stage of differentiation and become unable to undergo mitosis and replicate themselves further. For example, shortly after birth nerve cells (neurons) cease division and replication.

Despite there being no 'typical' cell, cells share certain characteristics. All have a cell membrane which encloses cytoplasm; in most cells, the cytoplasm surrounds a nucleus. (Mature red blood cells in humans do not have a nucleus, nevertheless they live for about 100 days.) Although the nucleus and cyto-plasm may be clearly distinguished using a light microscope to examine cells in slices of tissue (Chapter 1), to resolve finer detail an electron microscope may be used. As the wavelength of electrons is much shorter than light waves, electron microscopy can resolve structures about 1000 times smaller than the light microscope can. Within cytoplasm, electron microscopy reveals a range of membrane-bound organelles and other structures (Fig. 2.1) which carry out a variety of functions during the life of a cell. The term 'ultra-structure' is used to describe structures revealed by electron microscopy. A brief survey of the ultrastructure of cells in relation to their function is given below.

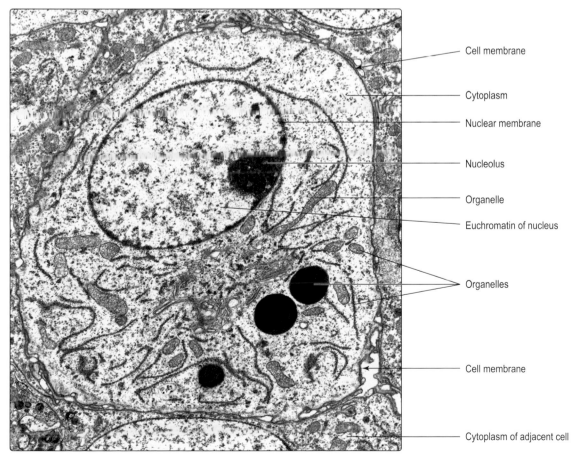

Cell membrane

Cytoplasm

Nuclear membrane

Nucleolus

Organelle

Euchromatin of nucleus

Organelles

Cell membrane

Cytoplasm of adjacent cell

Fig. 2.1 **Electron micrograph of a cell.** Low magnification.

Ultrastructure of cells and extracellular matrix

Cell membrane

All cells are surrounded by a cell (plasma) membrane, and its integrity is essential for the life of the cell. The cell membrane is a double-layered lipid–protein structure which has specific molecules embedded in it at intervals: the type of molecule(s) varies with the function of the cell. Most of the organelles within cells are surrounded by a similar lipid–protein membrane.

The cell membrane is semi-permeable and allows inward and outward passage of selected substances. It also forms an essential barrier to the exterior and a boundary for the internal structure of the cell. It may be involved in attachments to adjacent cells (see below) and in recognition and communication within and outside the cell. Within, it may communicate with its cytoplasm and some signals may pass to the nucleus. Outside, it may communicate with other 'self' cells, both normal and abnormal (e.g. tumour cells or virally infected cells). Many cells interact, via their cell membrane, with microbes, and various molecules foreign to the body and a variety of cellular activities are stimulated or inhibited as a result.

Nucleus and nucleolus

The nucleus contains the vast majority of the DNA of the cell. The DNA is the hereditary material that has the genetic code expressed in a double strand of DNA in each chromosome. (Chromosomes contain proteins as well as DNA.) The number of chromosomes in a typical cell is species specific (humans have 46). Human chromosomes comprise 22 homologous pairs and a pair of sex chromosomes (two X chromosomes in females and an X and a Y chromosome in males). One of each pair of chromosomes is derived from the mother's oocyte and the other from the father's spermatozoon (see, respectively, Chapters 16 and 15). The nucleus may also contain the structural and molecular mechanisms for the synthesis of RNA in one or more nucleoli.

The nucleus is enclosed by a nuclear membrane which is formed by two plasma membranes. In places, the nuclear membrane is perforated by pores which allow transport of material to and from the nucleus. The outer nuclear membrane is continuous in places with some membranes in the cytoplasm, and molecules (e.g. proteins

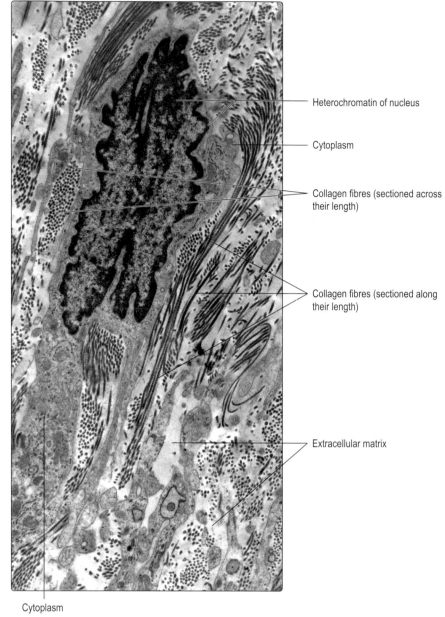

Cytoplasm

Fig. 2.2 **Electron micrograph of a cell.** Low magnification.

Labels on figure:
Heterochromatin of nucleus
Cytoplasm
Collagen fibres (sectioned across their length)
Collagen fibres (sectioned along their length)
Extracellular matrix

and RNA) travel between nucleus and cytoplasm by this route.

The appearance of nuclei varies in relation to their function. Individual chromosomes are not apparent in cells unless the cell is dividing. The nuclear material, comprising DNA, proteins and RNA, is known as chromatin and two types are described, euchromatin and heterochromatin. Euchromatin appears less dense than heterochromatin (Figs 2.1 and 2.2). The DNA molecules in euchromatin are uncoiled and are being used as coding for RNA synthesis which, in turn, directs protein synthesis in the cytoplasm. A large amount of euchromatin in a nucleus (Fig. 2.1) indicates that a wide variety of RNA molecules are being made (and types of protein produced as a result). In contrast, in

heterochromatin the DNA molecules are coiled and condensed and appear dense. The DNA in heterochromatin is mostly inactive, i.e. not directing the synthesis of RNA.

One or more nucleoli also appear as densely stained regions in the nuclei of cells actively synthesising proteins: their position may appear central or peripheral (Fig. 2.1). RNA molecules synthesised in the nucleolus leave the nucleus, via pores in the nuclear membrane, and are involved in organising protein synthesis in the cytoplasm.

Cytoplasm

Cytoplasm comprises a fluid matrix, a cytoskeleton, various membrane-bound organelles and may include stored molecules.

Cytoskeleton

The cytoskeleton of cells has several types of structure which affect the shape of the cells, e.g. tubular structures (centrosomes and microtubules) and protein filaments (intermediate and thin).

- *Centrosomes* (Fig. 2.3). These contain paired units, known as centrioles, which are set at right angles to each other and which contain nine triplets of microtubules (see below). Centriole tubules anchor other microtubules.
- *Microtubules*. Some microtubules are straight and long and allow the passage of substances within the cell. Many microtubules are polarised, i.e. they have specific ends with one end usually attached to a centrosome. Microtubules in some nerve cells transport molecules in a cytoplasmic

process which extends several centimetres (Chapter 6). Other microtubules assist in maintaining cell shape, compartmentalising the cytoplasm or facilitating movement of organelles within the cytoplasm. Microtubules are present in cilia, and in cells undergoing division (see below).
- *Intermediate filaments*. The main role of this group of filaments involves resisting external stresses on the cytoplasm by their attachment to specific internal cell structures. They include the protein keratin in the epithelium of skin (Chapter 7).
- *Thin (micro) filaments*. These filaments are formed from the protein actin. Actin filaments are present in most cells and are involved in moving organelles within cells, in cell movement, and exocytosis and endocytosis (see below). One specific role of actin in muscle cells involves interaction with thicker protein filaments of myosin, which results in muscle contraction (Chapter 5).

Cytoplasmic organelles

The main cytoplasmic organelles are mitochondria, endoplasmic reticulum, Golgi apparatus, vesicles and lysosomes. These organelles are involved in provi-

sion of energy for cellular processes, synthesis and secretion of protein, carbohydrate and lipid-based molecules, storage of proteins and degradation of waste material.

Mitochondria

Mitochondria vary in shape but many are ovoid (Figs 2.4 and 2.5). They are surrounded by an outer and inner membrane and provide most of the energy needs of the cell. The outer membrane is a typical plasma membrane, but the inner membrane has numerous infoldings known as cristae. These folds increase the surface area inside each mitochondrion and provide a matrix in which metabolic processes occur. The matrix comprises a viscous fluid containing enzymes associated with the tricarboxylic acid (TCA) cycle. Mitochondria are involved in oxidative phosphorylation, which results in the production of adenosine triphosphate (ATP). ATP acts as a store of energy that is used for various cell activities. Mitochondria contain very small amounts of DNA in the matrix which code for some mitochondrial proteins.

Endoplasmic reticulum

Endoplasmic reticulum is a membrane system similar in appearance to the plasma membrane. It is double layered

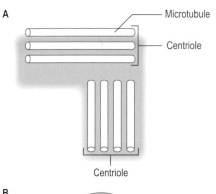
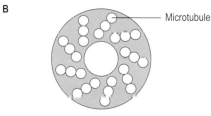

Fig. 2.3 **The structure of centrosomes sectioned (A) longitudinally through the paired centrioles (only some of the microtubules are in the plane of this diagram) and (B) a centriole sectioned transversely.**

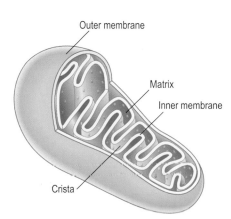

Fig. 2.4 **A cut open mitochondrion and its three-dimensional structure.**

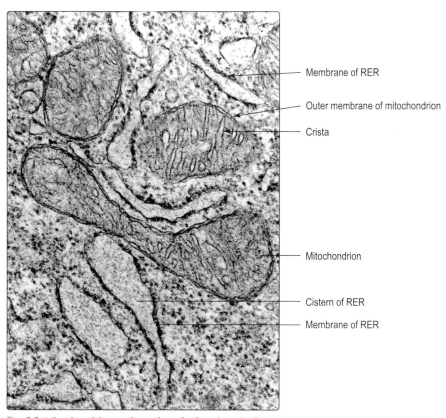

Fig. 2.5 **Mitochondrion and rough endoplasmic reticulum (RER).** Electron micrograph of part of a cell. Medium magnification.

and encloses a space known as a cistern (Fig. 2.5). In cells actively synthesising molecules, the cistern may be relatively wide. All membranes in the cytoplasm of a cell are probably linked and some link to the nuclear membrane. Two types of endoplasmic reticulum are described according to their appearance in electron micrographs.

- *Smooth endoplasmic reticulum (SER).* These membranes appear smooth and are sparse in cells except those synthesising lipids such as steroid hormones (Chapters 14–16). In some muscle cells, SER is especially important as it moves calcium ions which are essential for muscle contraction (Chapter 5).
- *Rough endoplasmic reticulum (RER).* These membranes appear rough (Fig. 2.5) as they are studded with ribosomes (see below). They are particularly prominent in cells synthesising proteins for export from the cell. Some proteins synthesised on RER are passed to the Golgi apparatus for further processing (see below).
  - Ribosomes are electron-dense structures containing RNA; some are attached to the membranes of RER

(Fig. 2.5), others lie free or form clusters in the cytoplasm (Fig. 2.6). Specific proteins are synthesised by ribosomes from amino acids. The specificity is determined by coded RNA arriving from the DNA in the nucleus. In general, proteins produced on RER are for export and those produced by free ribosomes are for internal use.

Vesicles, endocytosis and exocytosis

Membrane-bound vesicles are usually spherical. Many are involved in taking substances into and out of cells by the processes of endocytosis and exocytosis respectively (Fig. 2.6). It is usual to distinguish two types of endocytosis: pinocytosis involves the uptake of fluid and phagocytosis the uptake of solids (but fluid may enter in the same vesicle). In addition, the process of endocytosis may be non-specific or specific. In non-specific endocytosis the cell membrane becomes invaginated and then encloses some extracellular material. Specific endocytosis involves receptor molecules on the cell membrane that are able to bind specific (target) molecules. In specific endocytosis only the part of the cell membrane with the receptor molecules

(and their bound target molecules) invaginates and takes in the bound molecules; this process is known as receptor-mediated endocytosis (Fig. 2.6). The fate of endocytotic vesicles varies; some may fuse with lysosomes (see below) or the contents may have a specific use within the cell. Exocytosis is the process by which the contents of membrane-bound vesicles are released from a cell. The membrane around the vesicle fuses with the cell membrane and the contents of the vesicle are released from the cell (Fig. 2.6).

Golgi apparatus

The Golgi apparatus involves a stack of several parallel membranes (lying close to RER) and small membrane-bound vesicles (Fig. 2.6). Newly synthesised proteins pass in vesicles from RER to the Golgi membranes. The proteins (in vesicles) then pass between the layers of Golgi membranes. During the time spent in the Golgi apparatus various carbohydrate molecules may be added to the newly synthesised proteins. Vesicles leaving the Golgi stack may move towards the cell membrane and discharge their contents by exocytosis or release them for internal use; others

Fig. 2.6 **Endocytosis, exocytosis, and function of rough endoplasmic reticulum (RER), Golgi and lysosomes.** Arrows (within the cell) indicate movement of structures as the various functions occur.

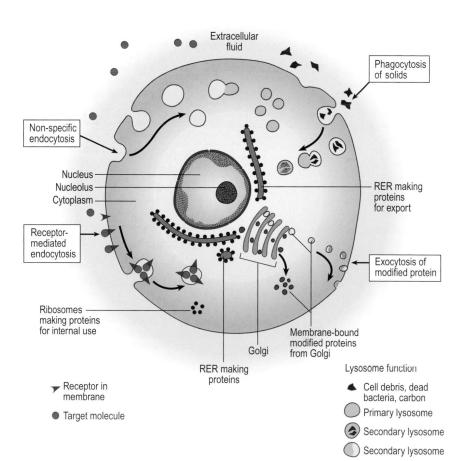

may remain stored in vesicles in the cell until they are needed.

Lysosomes
Lysosomes are membrane-bound organelles (Fig. 2.6) which are usually electron dense and thus appear dark in electron micrographs. They are formed via Golgi bodies and contain hydrolytic enzymes which are active at low (acidic) pH (e.g. acid phosphatases). Newly formed lysosomes are known as primary lysosomes and they may remain in a cell for some time before they become active. Lysosomes function by fusing with some endocytotic vesicles, other organelles or fragments of organelles, or other material; at this stage they become secondary lysosomes (Fig. 2.6). Lysosomal enzymes are released onto the ingested material and break down most of the molecules they contained. The small molecules formed as a result may be reused by the cell; other substances which resist digestion (e.g. carbon) remain in the lysosome. The integrity of the membrane around lysosomes is important as it ensures that the hydrolytic lysosomal enzymes do not pass into the cytoplasm and destroy the cell itself.

Cytoplasmic processes
The cytoplasm of some cells forms specific processes which extend from the cells. These are microvilli, cilia and flagella.

■ *Microvilli* (Fig. 2.7) project as finger-like cytoplasmic extensions from many epithelial cells, e.g. from the apical surface of cells lining some gut tubes and others lining some tubules in the kidney. Actin microfilaments in microvilli help maintain their shape. The microvilli increase the area of cell membrane in contact with the contents of the tube and this aids absorption of molecules from the tube into the cell.
■ *Cilia* are cytoplasmic processes which extend from the cell membranes of some epithelial cells, e.g. cells in the epithelium lining tubes transporting air to the lungs. Cilia are usually wider and longer than microvilli. Cilia have microtubules extending along their length which have a symmetrical arrangement. The microtubules are in a 9 + 2 pattern, which is apparent when sectioned across their length

(Fig. 2.8). The tubules are involved in moving the cilia in a regular, synchronised beat which propels the material on the surface of the ciliated cells in a particular direction (Chapter 11).
■ *Flagella* are similar to cilia and have symmetrically arranged microtubules but are much longer and wider than cilia. In humans, the only cells which have a flagellum are spermatozoa (the male gametes). Each spermatozoon is propelled by the beating of its flagellum as it travels the length of the female reproductive tract after copulation (Chapters 15 and 16).

Molecules stored in cytoplasm
Carbohydrates and lipids are stored in cytoplasm; most are not enclosed by a membrane. Glycogen is stored in many cells and acts as an energy reserve. It appears as dense particles in electron micrographs, some of which are clustered together and may occupy extensive regions of the cytoplasm. Lipids are stored in some cells generally as spherical masses. Some stored lipids act as precursor molecules for the synthesis of steroid hormones, others provide energy reserves. Proteins and glycoproteins are usually stored in membrane-bound vesicles and their contents discharged by exocytosis when needed.

Intercellular junctions
There are three specialised ways in which adjacent cells are attached to each other (Fig. 2.9).

■ *Tight junctions (zona occludens)*. In these junctions a short length of the outer cell membrane layers of adjacent cells is fused. These junctions prevent molecules from passing in between cells.

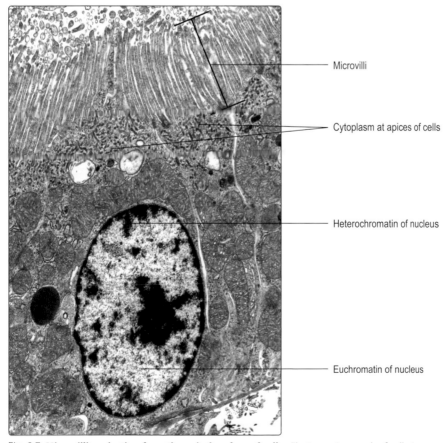

Fig. 2.7 **Microvilli projecting from the apical surface of cells.** Electron micrograph of cells. Low magnification.

Microvilli
Cytoplasm at apices of cells
Heterochromatin of nucleus
Euchromatin of nucleus

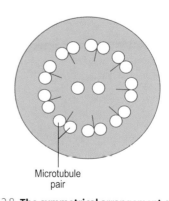

Microtubule pair

Fig. 2.8 **The symmetrical arrangement of microtubules (nine pairs + two) in a cilium sectioned across its length.**

- *Desmosomes (macula and zonula adherens).* These junctions are points (maculae) or encircling bands (zonulae) which appear in electron micrographs as dense regions between adjacent cell membranes. On the inside of the cell membrane in the region of a desmosome there is a dense plaque and components of the cytoskeleton. Desmosomes provide firm physical attachments between cells but do not prevent molecules moving in between the cells.
  - Hemidesmosomes are similar to desmosomes, but they are one sided; the cell membrane interacts with extracellular material.
- *Gap junctions.* At these junctions membranes from adjacent cells are closely applied but they are not fused. Gap junctions allow the passage of ions and very small molecules from one cell to an adjacent cell. They are particularly important between heart muscle cells as ion movement between such cells is an essential part of coordinating contraction of heart muscle (Chapter 10).

Extracellular matrix

Many cells are adjacent to extracellular matrix and some are entirely surrounded by it. Extracellular matrix varies in form and function in different parts of the body (Chapter 4). Some proteins (e.g. collagen) form fibres in extracellular matrix, and their appearance depends on the angle at which they are sectioned (Fig. 2.2).

The cell cycle and cell division

The cell cycle is the series of stages through which a cell passes between successive rounds of the cell division process known as mitosis (Fig. 2.10). The actual event of mitosis takes a relatively short time in the cycle, sometimes less than an hour. The stages a cell passes through before successive mitotic divisions are collectively known as interphase and take considerably longer (several hours or days). During interphase, events occur which may relate to the specific functions of the cell, e.g. protein synthesis and secretion. A cell in interphase must also undergo specific processes to replicate its DNA in preparation for mitosis.

The interphase of the cell cycle is divided into three stages (Fig. 2.10). After

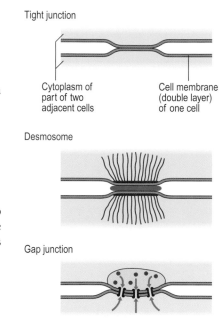

Fig. 2.9 **The structure of cell junctions.** Blue arrows show the passages along which ions travel in gap junctions.

mitosis, cells enter the G_1 phase, which is often the longest phase of the cycle. During G_1, cells synthesise many molecules, increase the volume of the cytoplasm and increase the number of organelles. These synthetic processes may be specific for a cell to carry out its functions as well as to produce molecules necessary for the next phase. At the end of G_1, the cells move into the next phase (the S phase) when they begin to synthesise new DNA. During the S phase the new DNA is assembled along the length of the existing double strand of DNA in each chromosome by the process of base pairing; this duplicates the existing DNA. At the end of the S phase, instead of a double strand of DNA in each chromosome there are four strands of DNA (arranged as two chromatids). When DNA replication is completed, the cells move into the G_2 phase, which is when the cell prepares for mitosis. The G_2 phase is usually much shorter than the G_1 phase.

A cell which undergoes a mitotic cell division becomes two identical offspring cells with the same number of chromosomes containing the same amount and type of DNA as the original cell. Mitosis may be described in five stages.

- *Prophase.* During this stage the DNA in chromosomes becomes very coiled and condensed and appears as very dense chromatin. The nucleolus disappears and RNA production ceases. Towards the end of prophase (Fig. 2.11A) chromosomes appear as

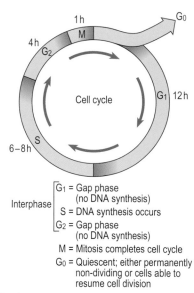

Fig. 2.10 **The phases of the cell cycle.**

two parallel chromatids joined at a point known as the centromere. Each chromatid contains an old strand of DNA and the newly synthesised copy strand. At this time, the centrosome of the cell has been duplicated and they move to opposite poles of the cell. Part of each centrosome begins to give rise to an array of microtubules which will form a mitotic spindle (see below).

- *Prometaphase.* This stage begins with the disappearance of the nuclear membrane. During this phase chromosomes are still randomly arranged in the cytoplasm. A mitotic spindle forms and each chromosome begins to move towards the microtubules at the equator of the spindle.
- *Metaphase.* In this stage (Fig. 2.11B) each chromosome attaches (by its centromere) at a separate point on the equator of the spindle, an arrangement described as forming a metaphase plate. Such plates are readily visible with the light microscope in actively dividing cells.
- *Anaphase.* During anaphase the chromosomes split along their length separating the two chromatids which then move away from each other and towards opposite poles of the spindle (Fig. 2.11C). The separation of the chromatids follows the track of the microtubules of the spindle. Towards the end of anaphase a depression begins to develop around

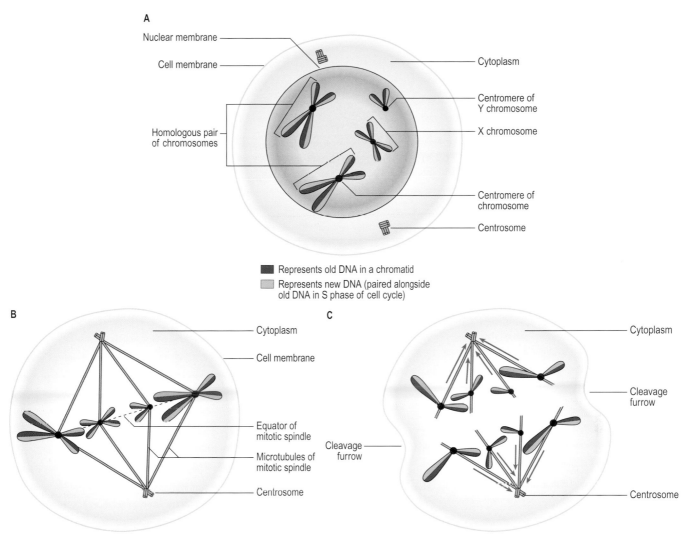

A

Nuclear membrane

Cell membrane

Homologous pair
of chromosomes

Cytoplasm

Centromere of
Y chromosome

X chromosome

Centromere of
chromosome

Centrosome

■ Represents old DNA in a chromatid
□ Represents new DNA (paired alongside
old DNA in S phase of cell cycle)

B

Cytoplasm

Cell membrane

Equator of
mitotic spindle

Microtubules of
mitotic spindle

Centrosome

C

Cytoplasm

Cleavage
furrow

Cleavage
furrow

Centrosome

Fig. 2.11 **(A) Late prophase, (B) metaphase and (C) anaphase stages of mitosis.** Only one pair of homologous chromosomes (of the 22 pairs in humans) and an X and a Y chromosome are shown. In (C) arrows show the direction of movement of the chromatids.

the cytoplasm and it is known as the cleavage furrow.

■ *Telophase*. The chromatids reach the opposite poles of the spindle and the spindle disappears. The furrow in the cytoplasm deepens and splits the cytoplasm as cell membranes appear between the two new offspring cells, a process known as cytokinesis (Fig. 2.12). Each new cell contains chromatids (each containing double-stranded DNA) which are exact copies of the DNA in the original chromosome. Each chromatid is now a new chromosome. These chromosomes uncoil and appear as chromatin as a nuclear membrane develops, surrounds the chromatin and reforms the nucleus.

On completion of the cell cycle, the two new cells may enter a G₁ phase and prepare for further rounds of the cycle.

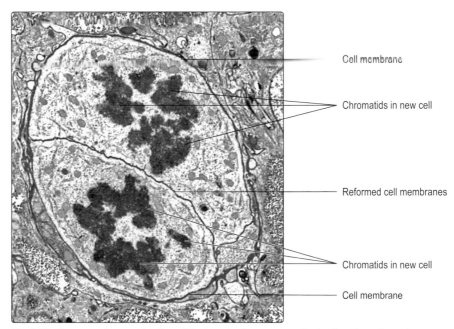

Cell membrane

Chromatids in new cell

Reformed cell membranes

Chromatids in new cell

Cell membrane

Fig. 2.12 **Electron micrograph of a cell in the telophase stage of mitosis.** The cell membrane has formed around each new cell and completed cytokinesis. The nuclear membrane has not yet reformed. Although all of the chromatids (i.e. new chromosomes) do not lie in the plane of section, they appear as densely stained clumps and have yet to uncoil. Low magnification.

Some cells may suspend their progression around the cell cycle (usually at the G_1 stage) and enter a G_0 phase (Fig. 2.10). Some cells in the G_0 phase may eventually re-enter the cycle and replicate themselves when, for example, they are needed to replace dead or damaged similar cells. Other cells halt their progression around the cycle, undergo differentiation and carry out specific functions before they die without having divided again.

Meiosis

Meiosis is a type of cell division in which the number of chromosomes (and DNA) in the offspring cells is half that in the parent cell. This occurs only in the formation of gametes, i.e. ova in females and spermatozoa in males. Meiosis ensures that on fertilisation the normal number of chromosomes (and their DNA content) is present in the fertilised ovum (the zygote). The process of meiosis ensures that there is a mixing of maternally and paternally derived chromosomes (and thus genes). This ensures diversity of the gene pool of a species. Further details of meiosis are described in Chapters 15 and 16.

Summary

- A cell is the basic unit of life formed from cytoplasm and a nucleus (in most cells) enclosed by a cell membrane.
- The nucleus contains DNA (in chromosomes), proteins and RNA.
- In non-dividing cells, nuclear contents are described as chromatin:
  - heterochromatin is densely stained and is largely inactive
  - euchromatin is palely stained as the DNA is uncoiled and coding RNA to direct protein synthesis
  - a nucleolus is present in nuclei of cells producing RNA.
- Cytoplasm contains organelles which carry out specific functions:
  - tubules and protein filaments give shape to cells and aid movement (of material in cells and of cells themselves)
  - mitochondria provide energy (ATP) for the cell
  - endoplasmic reticulum, which is formed from membranes surrounding a cistern, is involved in synthesis. RER has bound ribosomes and synthesises proteins mainly for export; SER is involved in lipid synthesis. Free ribosomes synthesise proteins mainly for internal use
  - membrane-bound vesicles are involved in uptake of substances into the cell (endocytosis) and export of substances (exocytosis)
  - the Golgi apparatus has membranes and vesicles and modifies synthesised proteins by adding, for example, carbohydrates
  - lysosomes are membrane bound and contain hydrolytic enzymes. Lysosomes fuse with endocytotic vesicles and digest their contents.
- Cytoplasm in some cells forms projections, for example cilia and microvilli, and may store carbohydrate, lipids or proteins.
- Specialised parts of cell membranes of adjacent cells form junctions which help to bind the cells together, prevent molecules moving in between the cells, or aid movement of ions between adjacent cells.
- Cell division (mitosis) occurs in many types of cell. Prior to mitosis, cells synthesise copy strands of their DNA in the S phase of the cell cycle:
  - In the prophase stage of mitosis chromosomes condense and become visible as individual units. A spindle forms of microtubules. Gradually, the nuclear membrane disappears and (at metaphase) the chromosomes move to the equator of the spindle and attach to the microtubules. In the next phase (anaphase) the chromosomes split along their length and each half moves towards a pole of the spindle. Mitosis ends with telophase as the spindle disappears and the nuclear membrane reforms and encloses the uncoiling chromosomes. The cytoplasm of the original cell splits and two new cells are formed with each having the same number of chromosomes (and amount of DNA) as the original cell.

Chapter 3
Primary tissues 1: epithelial tissue

Introduction to primary issues

The microscopic structures of the body were classified originally into four primary tissues:

- epithelial tissue
- connective tissue
- muscle tissue
- nerve tissue.

This classification is still in wide use and is the basis for all studies aimed at understanding the structure and function of normal and abnormal cells, tissues and organs of the body.

Epithelial tissues in general lie on surfaces (*epi* = on or upon) and many carry out secretory and other highly specialised functions. Cells from some epithelia migrate from surfaces during development in utero and form glands within the body (e.g. the pancreas) and produce and secrete various molecules. The names of the other primary tissues (connective, muscle and nerve) indicate the prime functions of the components of these tissues in their titles, respectively the connection of structures, contraction of muscles and conduction of nerve impulses.

Epithelial tissue

Epithelial tissue consists mainly of epithelial cells which form layers (epithelia) covering the body and structures in the body such as organs. Epithelial tissues also form the linings of hollow structures in the body and form the outer layer(s) of some membranes. Epithelial cells are the major cell type forming the parenchyma of some solid organs and glands and are involved in synthesising and secreting many substances. In addition to secretion, epithelia are involved in a variety of functions, including transport of substances, absorption of molecules, modulation of permeability and protection, and in detecting some sensations. Although epithelia exhibit a variety of forms and functions they all consist of epithelial cells which are tightly bound to each other by specialised junctions (Chapter 2). The importance of epithelia to body function is apparent when it is realised that every molecule or organism that enters (or leaves) the body has to pass through an epithelium.

Epithelia lining and covering structures

Epithelia are categorised as:

- *simple epithelia*, which consist of a single layer of epithelial cells

- *compound (stratified) epithelia*, which display several layers of cells.

In each of these categories there are sub-categories, classified according to the shape of the epithelial cells.

Simple epithelia

In simple epithelia, each epithelial cell is attached to a basement membrane (sometimes called a basal lamina). The basement membrane is a concentration of extracellular material, including glycoproteins and connective tissue fibres (mainly collagen) (Chapter 4).

Simple epithelia comprise four main types:

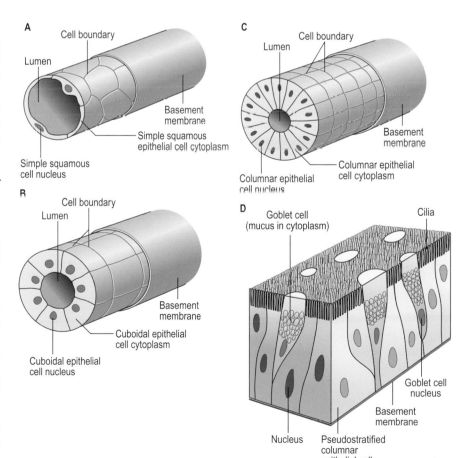

Fig. 3.1 **Simple epithelia.** (A) Simple squamous epithelium, (B) simple cuboidal epithelium, (C) simple columnar epithelium and (D) pseudostratified epithelium (with ciliated columnar epithelial cells and goblet cells).

- simple squamous
- simple cuboidal
- simple columnar
- pseudostratified columnar.

Simple squamous epithelia

Squamous epithelial cells are irregularly shaped, flattened (pavement like) and fit intimately together. The nuclei in squamous cells often occupy a central position, and, given that the cytoplasm of the cells is generally flattened, a bulge may be apparent in the region of the nucleus (Fig. 3.1A). An important function of simple, squamous epithelial cells is that they facilitate the transport of gases and/or other substances across the epithelium. Examples of the location of squamous epithelia include the linings of blood vessels (Fig. 3.2), which are known as endothelia, and the walls of lung alveoli, i.e. regions where the movement of oxygen and carbon dioxide is important.

Simple cuboidal epithelia

Epithelial cells in cuboidal epithelia are shaped like boxes, with fairly square profiles, and each cell has a roughly centrally placed nucleus. Unlike squamous cells, their nuclei do not bulge as there is ample cytoplasm around them (Fig. 3.1B). Examples of where this cell type may be found include the lining of the walls of ducts in the liver (Fig. 3.3) and the walls of ducts draining glands, e.g. sweat glands. Their function varies with their location and may involve synthesis and secretion, or excretion, or absorption of molecules.

Simple columnar epithelia

Columnar epithelial cells have the shape of columns with their longest dimension at right angles to the basement membrane. Their nuclei typically lie near the basement membrane (Fig. 3.1C) or about half-way along their length. Columnar epithelial cells are present in the lining of the wall of the gastrointestinal tract (Fig. 3.4), the gall bladder and some tubules in the kidney, for example. In many locations, they are associated with the function of absorption of substances into the cells across their apical (luminal) surface and then out of the cells via the basal surface and then across their basement membrane. The apical surfaces of many absorptive columnar epithelial cells display a 'brush border' appearance (Fig. 3.4) when examined by light microscopy and this is due to the presence of microvilli (Chapter 2). The microvilli increase

Connective tissue

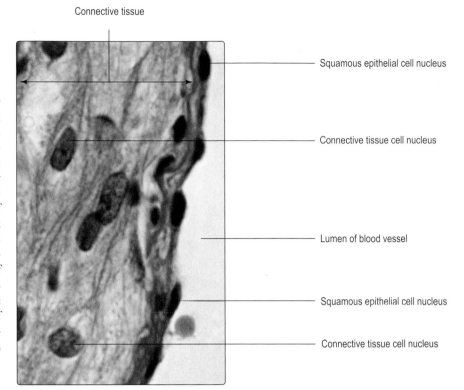

Squamous epithelial cell nucleus

Connective tissue cell nucleus

Lumen of blood vessel

Squamous epithelial cell nucleus

Connective tissue cell nucleus

Fig. 3.2 **Simple squamous epithelium, lining a blood vessel.** The squamous cells lining blood vessels are known as endothelial cells; they may appear so flattened that it is not possible to distinguish the extent of the cytoplasm (even at this magnification). The nuclei may appear to protrude into the lumen with no intervening cytoplasm. Adjacent connective tissue supports the endothelium. Very high magnification.

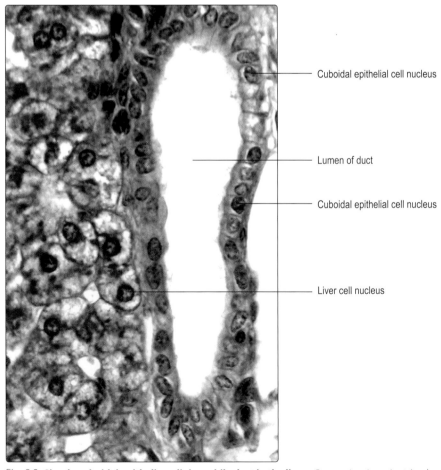

Cuboidal epithelial cell nucleus

Lumen of duct

Cuboidal epithelial cell nucleus

Liver cell nucleus

Fig. 3.3 **Simple cuboidal epithelium, lining a bile duct in the liver.** Connective tissue is stained blue. Special stain. High magnification.

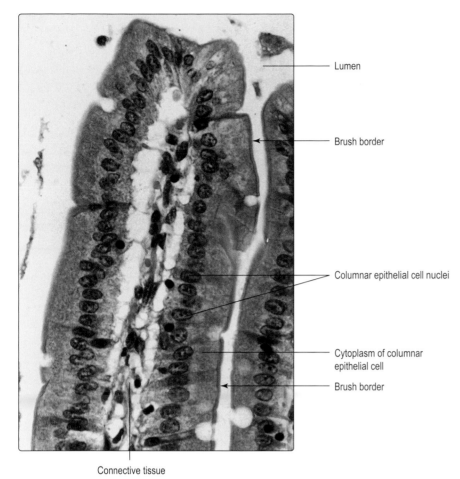

Connective tissue

Fig. 3.4 **Simple columnar epithelium, lining the small intestine.** The cytoplasm of columnar epithelial cells, sectioned along their length, extends beyond their nuclei towards the apical (luminal) surface. In some cells, the apical surface displays a brush border. High magnification.

the surface area of the luminal membrane of absorptive cells and thus increase the efficiency of the transport of molecules.

Pseudostratified columnar epithelia

This type of epithelium is called 'pseudostratified' because it appears as though it is composed of several layers but each cell actually has an attachment to the basement membrane (Fig. 3.1D). The appearance of stratification is because the nuclei in the various cells in the epithelium are located at different levels in relation to the basement membrane and a single section through the cells does not usually display the whole extent of their cytoplasm. This type of epithelium lines much of the respiratory tract (Fig. 3.5). Specialised epithelial cells are present in this 'respiratory' epithelium; some produce mucus (unicellular glands known as goblet cells) and others have cytoplasmic projections on their luminal surface known as cilia (Chapter 2). Together, cilia and mucus entrap solid particles, e.g. dust and bacteria. The cilia move in a synchronised beat, a bit like

a whiplash, and this moves the mucus and its contents. The general direction of flow of the mucus is away from the lungs and towards the pharynx where most is swallowed.

Compound (stratified) epithelia

Compound (stratified) epithelia are composed of several layers of cells. Only cells in the deepest layer are attached to the basement membrane. Sub-categories are classified according to the shape of the surface epithelial cells:

- stratified squamous
- stratified cuboidal
- stratified columnar
- transitional.

Stratified squamous epithelia

Stratified squamous epithelia have layers of cells of cuboidal or columnar shape but the surface cells are squamous (flattened and pavement like). Typical regions of the body where stratified squamous epithelia are present include the linings of the oesophagus, vagina (Fig. 3.6) and anal canal where the epithelia provide some physical protection

from abrasion. The squamous surface cells are shed, especially when abrasion occurs, but they are replaced by deeper cells which become flattened as they move to the surface layer. Cells located at the base of the epithelium are the progenitor (stem) cells for the rest of the epithelial cells. Mitosis of these stem cells ensures that the layers of cells are constantly replaced as some new cells migrate to the surface. Importantly, some cells remain in the basal layer and continue to function as stem cells.

The cells in a specialised type of stratified squamous epithelium produce the protein keratin. The epithelium of the skin, known as the epidermis, is the main region of the body where this type of epithelium is present and it is categorised as a keratinised, stratified, squamous epithelium (Fig. 3.7). The keratin produced by the epithelial cells (keratinocytes) fills the cells in the upper layers of the epidermis and these cells become flattened and they die. Keratin from the dead cells forms the surface layers of the skin and it gradually flakes off (desquamates). Keratin makes the skin waterproof, reduces water loss by evaporation, provides protection from abrasion, and resists the penetration of the skin by many molecules and microorganisms.

Stratified cuboidal epithelia

The surface cells of stratified cuboidal epithelia are cuboidal in shape and usually only two layers are present. This type of epithelium lines ducts draining some glands, e.g. salivary glands.

Stratified columnar epithelia

This type of epithelium is present in only a few locations in the body, e.g. some large ducts and portions of the male urethra. Its deepest layer is typically low cuboidal and the surface cells are columnar in shape.

Transitional epithelium

This type of epithelium is a highly specialised stratified epithelium present only in the regions of the body in contact with urine. Transitional epithelium lines parts of the kidney, the ureters, the urinary bladder (Fig. 3.8) and parts of the urethra (Chapter 13). A key function of transitional epithelium is its ability to act as a permeability barrier between hypertonic urine and isotonic tissue fluid and blood. In addition, the transitional epithelium lining the bladder is able to stretch as the bladder distends and stores urine. The appearance of transitional epithelium depends on the

Fig. 3.5 **Pseudostratified columnar epithelium lining the respiratory tract.** The nuclei of the epithelial cells appear to be in layers. The cytoplasm of goblet cells is relatively palely stained as they are filled with carbohydrates which do not react strongly with haematoxylin and eosin. The luminal surface of ciliated columnar cells appears fragmented and can be distinguished from the surface of epithelial cells with microvilli (cf. Fig. 3.4). High magnification.

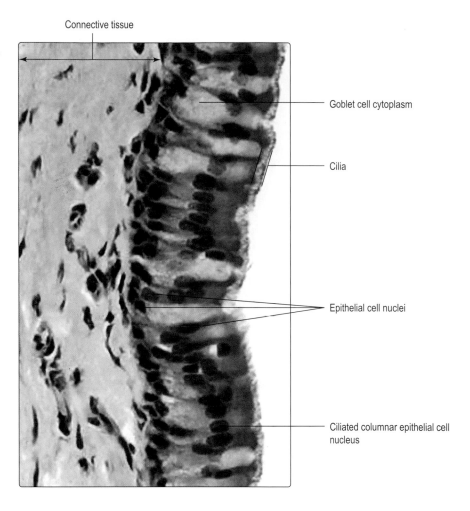

Connective tissue

Goblet cell cytoplasm

Cilia

Epithelial cell nuclei

Ciliated columnar epithelial cell nucleus

Fig. 3.6 **Stratified squamous epithelium lining the vagina.** The cells in surface layers are squamous. Their nuclei appear elongated and the cytoplasm sparse if they are sectioned across their narrowest dimension. Medium magnification.

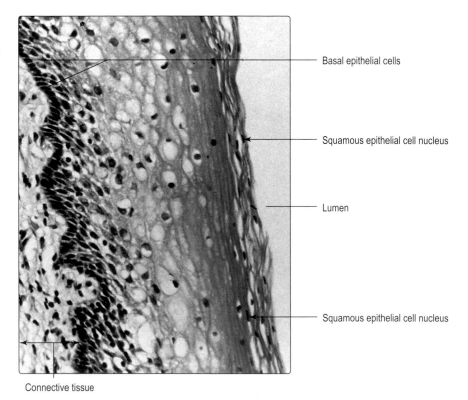

Basal epithelial cells

Squamous epithelial cell nucleus

Lumen

Squamous epithelial cell nucleus

Connective tissue

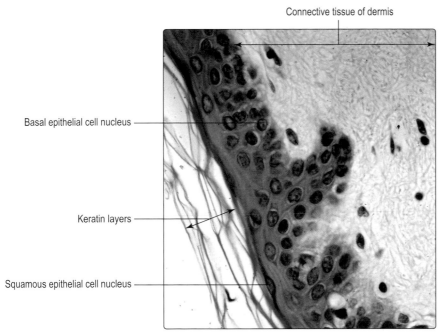

Fig. 3.7 **Keratinised, stratified, squamous epithelium of (thin) skin.** The surface layers consist of the protein keratin. Cells just below the keratin are squamous. Cells in the basal layers are cuboidal. High magnification.

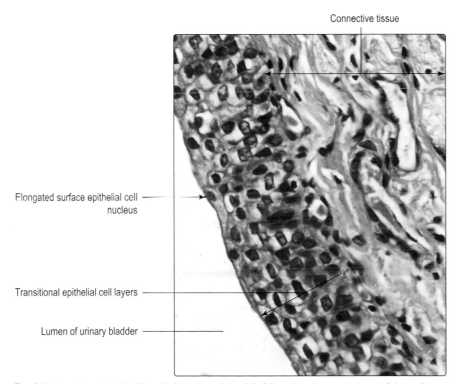

Fig. 3.8 **Transitional epithelium lining the urinary bladder.** The elongated shape of the surface epithelial cells in this layered epithelium indicates that the bladder was partially inflated when it was fixed. High magnification.

amount it is stretched. In an empty bladder, numerous epithelial cell layers are apparent. As the volume of urine in the bladder increases, the surface epithelial cells become flattened and the number of layers of cells reduced, but, importantly, they continue to function as a permeability barrier.

Epithelial glands and membranes

Glands
Epithelial gland cells are highly specialised and synthesise molecules for secretion which may be protein, carbohydrate or lipid based. Epithelial gland cells may form the major components of organs,

e.g. the liver and salivary glands, or relatively small components of other structures, e.g. sweat glands of the skin.

There are two main functional types of gland in the body:

■ *exocrine glands* that secrete their products onto epithelial surfaces via ducts
■ *endocrine glands* that secrete their products (hormones) directly into blood vessels.

Other secretory gland cells are present in the body. Some, known as paracrine glands, secrete factors into adjacent regions, and unicellular glands such as goblet cells secrete mucus onto the surfaces of the gastrointestinal and the respiratory tract (Fig. 3.5), for example.

Structurally, exocrine glands are of two types: simple or compound. Simple glands are drained by a single, unbranched duct and the secretory cells forming the gland may be arranged as straight or coiled tubules or in a spherical arrangement described as 'acinar' (Fig. 3.9A,B,C, respectively). Compound glands have a branching duct system that carries the secretion from gland cells arranged as tubules or acini or a combination of the two (Fig. 3.9D).

Exocrine glands synthesise their secretory products and may store them in membrane-bound structures. Secretions are released from the cells by three mechanisms:

■ *merocrine secretion* (Fig. 3.10A) involves exocytosis (Chapter 2) of the product, which is typically protein based, and constitutes the commonest arrangement; the pancreas secretes pancreatic enzymes by this method
■ *apocrine secretion* (Fig. 3.10B) involves the release of membrane-bound vesicles of secretory product from the apex of the cell; this arrangement is associated, mainly, with lipid-based products as secreted by some sweat glands and the modified sweat glands that form the mammary glands
■ *holocrine secretion* (Fig. 3.10C) involves the breakdown and release of the contents of the whole cell; sebaceous glands of skin utilise this mode of secretion (Chapter 7).

Release of secretion from exocrine glands may be enhanced by nervous or hormonal stimuli acting on specialised cells known as myoepithelial cells. These

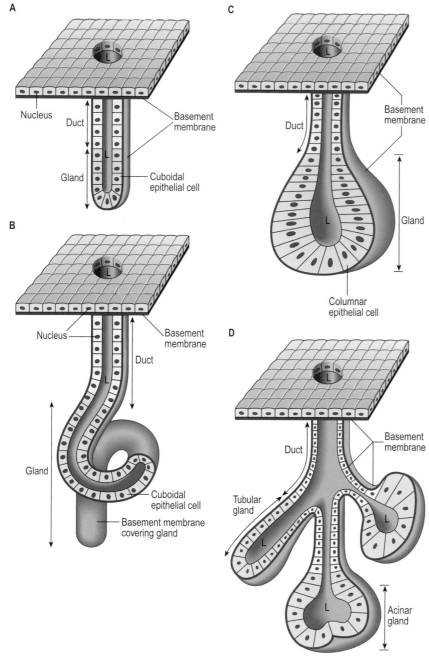

specialised epithelial cells surround the secretory units (e.g. acini) and they contain contractile proteins similar to those in muscle cells. Under nervous or hormonal stimulation, the contractile proteins in myoepithelial cells contract and this applies pressure to the secretory units and helps to expel their secretions.

Membranes

Epithelia form the surface layers of many membranes in the body, e.g. serous membranes. Serous membranes are very thin and their epithelia are usually supported by sparse connective tissue. Serous epithelial cells are usually cuboidal or squamous in shape and form a simple epithelium, and they secrete small amounts of fluid onto the surface of the membrane. Serous membranes have a variety of functions, including covering organs and supporting the blood vessels and nerves passing to them. Some serous membranes form double-layered structures and the inner visceral layer covering an organ is continuous with an outer (parietal) layer. The two layers are continuous and enclose a fluid-filled space. This arrangement of serous membranes is particularly important for organs which move as they function, e.g. each lung is enveloped by serous visceral and parietal pleural membranes which enclose the pleural cavity, the heart is enveloped by pericardial membranes enclosing the pericardial cavity, and parts of the gastrointestinal tract are enveloped by peritoneal membranes which enclose the peritoneal cavity.

Fig. 3.9 **Exocrine gland structure.** (A) Simple tubular gland, (B) simple coiled tubular gland, (C) simple acinar gland and (D) compound tubuloacinar gland. L, lumen.

Recognising epithelia, other primary tissues and organs

If cells are lining or covering a surface it will give the first clue as to whether these are epithelial cells forming an epithelium. To categorise the type of epithelium, the number of layers of cells and the shape of the cells must be determined and this is easier at higher magnifications at which it is usually possible to identify individual cell nuclei and their cytoplasm.

Connective tissue connects the basement membranes of epithelia to other structures and is thus readily recognised if an epithelium has been identified.

- In skin, the epithelium (epidermis) is adjacent to the connective tissue of the dermis (Fig. 3.7).

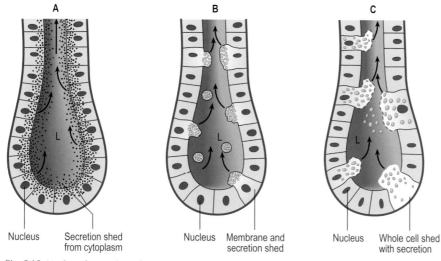

Fig. 3.10 **Modes of secretion of exocrine glands.** (A) Merocrine, (B) apocrine and (C) holocrine. L, lumen.

- In many tubes, e.g. of the digestive (Fig. 3.4), respiratory (Fig. 3.5), reproductive (Fig. 3.6) and urinary (Fig. 3.8) systems, the epithelia and basement membranes are adjacent to connective tissue (known as the lamina propria). The epithelium, basement membrane and connective tissue lamina propria together are described as a mucous membrane (a mucosa). The epithelial surfaces of such structures are kept moist by glandular secretions which are usually mucus or, in the case of the urinary tract, by urine. In addition,

smooth muscle (the muscularis mucosae) lies deep to the mucosa of some of these tubes.
- In blood vessels, the squamous epithelium (endothelium) is adjacent to connective tissue (Fig. 3.2) and, in some vessels, smooth muscle cells are also in close proximity.

Connective tissue occurs in regions other than adjacent to epithelia; further details which aid recognising primary tissues, other than epithelia, are given in Chapters 4–6.

Recognising organs relies on determining the primary tissues present and their arrangement. The liver is a multifunctional organ in which epithelial gland cells (hepatocytes) make up the majority of the organ, the parenchyma (Figs 3.3 and 3.11). Connective tissue (known as stroma) is also present and it provides support for, and connects, the hepatocytes, blood vessels and ducts in the gland. Knowing the normal arrangement of the cells and tissues in an organ is essential before being able to decide whether abnormalities are present.

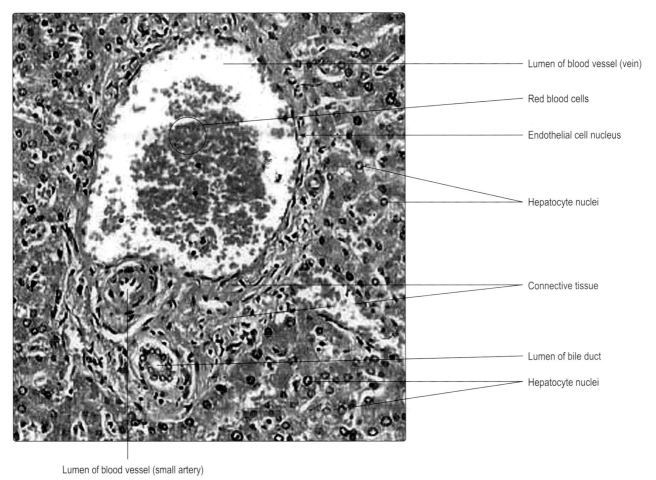

Fig. 3.11 **Liver.** Epithelial gland cells (hepatocytes) form the major component (the parenchyma) of this organ. The hepatocytes, blood vessels and ducts (draining bile) are supported and connected by connective tissue (stroma). A cuboidal epithelium lines the bile duct and endothelial cells line the blood vessels. (Connective tissue is more readily distinguished with special stains; see Fig. 3.3.) Medium magnification.

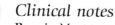

Clinical notes

Repair Most types of epithelia are constantly being renewed under normal circumstances by mitosis of undifferentiated stem cells in the epithelium, e.g. the life span of epithelial cells lining parts of the gut tube is less than a week. Most damaged epithelia are able to repair themselves by the mitotic activity of their stem cells and the rate at which this happens can readily be seen as cut skin repairs.

Tumours Many tumours in humans arise from epithelial cells undergoing abnormally high levels of cell proliferation when new cells produced by mitosis exceed the rate at which cells are lost. If the new growth of epithelial cells remains localised, it forms a benign tumour; if the new epithelial cells penetrate the basement membrane, the growth is malignant and known as a carcinoma. It is only after this invasion through the basement membrane has occurred that cancerous cells can spread to distant sites in the process known as metastasis. The extent to which cancerous epithelial cells have penetrated their basement membrane and have changed their appearance is used to judge the invasiveness of the tumour.

Summary

Epithelial tissue consists of epithelial cells attached to each other:

- A simple epithelium has a single layer of epithelial cells and each is attached to the basement membrane.
- A compound (stratified) epithelium has several layers of epithelial cells and only those in the basal layer are attached to the basement membrane.
- Epithelial cells line or cover structures in the body, form some membranes and form glands which secrete a variety of molecules:
  - exocrine glands discharge their secretions onto surfaces
  - endocrine glands discharge their secretions into blood vessels
  - paracrine and unicellular glands discharge their secretions in their local area.

Epithelial tissue has a variety of functions, reflected in its structure:

- secretion
- absorption
- modulation of permeability to molecules
- physical protection
- detection of some sensations.

Chapter 4
Primary tissues 2: connective tissue

All connective tissues consist of cells derived from the mesoderm layer of the embryo (see Mitchell B, Sharma R. *Embryology: An Illustrated Colour Text.* Elsevier: 2004). In most types of connective tissue the cells are widely spaced and separated by extracellular matrix which they have synthesised and secreted. The types of cell and the components and consistency of the extracellular matrix relate to the location and function of the particular type of connective tissue.

Blood may be categorised as a connective tissue since its cells arise from mesoderm, but the extracellular matrix (plasma) is fluid (Chapter 8). Bone and cartilage are classified as connective tissues and they have an extracellular matrix that is relatively solid. In the case of bone, the matrix is mineralised with calcium salts which confer rigidity to the bone and the ability to resist deforming forces (Chapter 9).

Cell types in connective tissue (excluding blood, bone and cartilage)

The major cell type found in many connective tissues is the fibroblast. In many instances, fibroblasts are identified by their densely stained, elongated nuclei which do not appear to be associated with much cytoplasm (Figs 4.1 and 4.2). Fibroblasts secrete long, fibre-like protein molecules (e.g. collagen and elastin) and many of the other large molecules in the extracellular matrix.

If connective tissue is damaged, it may be repaired by the ability of fibroblasts to undergo mitosis and to synthesise new matrix. If fibroblasts are actively secreting matrix proteins, their appearance is changed: their nuclei are larger and relatively palely stained and nucleoli are apparent (Chapter 3, see Fig. 3.2). This appearance is a result of the activity of the DNA (and nucleolus) in the synthetic processes which produce new molecules for the extracellular matrix. (Convention-

ally, a cell with the suffix 'blast' indicates a rapidly dividing cell. However, in the case of the fibroblast, the term is usually reserved for the differentiated non-dividing cell, which might more appropriately be known as a fibrocyte.)

Several other types of cell occur in connective tissues; some are restricted to a particular type of connective tissue and others to the functional state of the tissue.

They are:

- *mast cells*, which store granules containing specific molecules (e.g. histamine). When released from mast cells these molecules modify the permeability of blood vessels as part of an inflammatory reaction (Chapter 8)

- *macrophages*, which are able to phagocytose and digest bacteria and cell debris. They are also able to phagocytose, but not digest, inert substances, e.g. carbon particles. In addition, they aid the immune response to antigens (Chapter 8)
- *white blood cells* and *plasma cells*, which may be in transit through the connective tissue or responding locally as part of an immune response (Chapter 8)
- *adipocytes*, which store fats (lipids) in their cytoplasm (Fig. 4.1). The fats may be metabolised and provide energy and various metabolites when needed. Adipocytes also provide insulation, give shape to the body and act as physical protection, e.g. around the kidney.

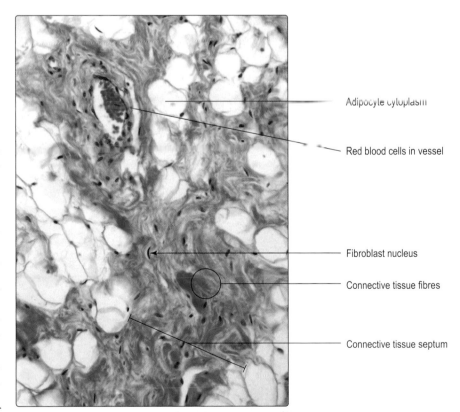

Adipocyte cytoplasm

Red blood cells in vessel

Fibroblast nucleus

Connective tissue fibres

Connective tissue septum

Fig. 4.1 **Connective tissue, fibroblasts, fibres and adipocytes.** Protein fibres, fibroblasts and extracellular matrix form septa between clusters of white adipocytes. The adipocytes appear empty as lipid which filled the cytoplasm has been extracted during histological processing. Red blood cells are present in an endothelium-lined blood vessel. Medium magnification.

Extracellular matrix of connective tissue

The extracellular matrix of connective tissue comprises ground substance and protein fibres. It is the combination of these two elements that is important in determining the function of the connective tissue.

Ground substance

Ground substance is a complex mixture of large molecules containing carbohydrates and protein, and tissue fluid containing water, salts, other small, soluble molecules and dissolved gases. The tissue fluid component ensures gases and nutrients move readily between blood vessels and connective tissue cells and other cells in the region. The large molecules (glycoproteins, proteoglycans and glycosoaminoglycans) bind the components of the extracellular matrix together altering the viscosity of the gel-like matrix and conferring on it different properties. In addition, the matrix molecules act as adhesion sites for various transient cell types which may be involved in immune responses.

Protein fibres

The protein fibres that are present in extracellular matrix of connective tissues are of two main types: collagen and elastin. Collagen is characterised by tensile strength and elastin by elasticity.

Collagen

Collagen is synthesised by fibroblasts and about 20 types have been identified but only a few are common. Different types of collagen are found in specific locations:

- types I and II collagen are in bone and skin (Fig. 4.2) and provide strength
- type II is in cartilage and provides strength and allows some distortion and recoil
- type III (known as reticulin) provides fine supporting fibres, e.g. for liver cells (Fig. 4.3)
- type IV is in basement membranes and provides firm attachments for epithelial cells (Fig. 4.4).

Elastin

Elastin molecules are also made and secreted by fibroblasts. The molecules may be formed into sheets (laminae) or distributed irregularly as fibres. Elastin molecules are predominantly in parts of the body where deformation and reformation occurs. Elastin is present in skin and in the walls of arteries (Fig. 4.5). Some arteries are distended as blood is pumped into them and then they recoil (owing to the elastin fibres recoiling), thus ensuring the blood continues to flow (Chapter 10).

Connective tissue types

Connective tissues may be divided into three major types (excluding bone, cartilage and blood):

- connective tissue 'proper' is also described as generalised connective tissue and is subdivided into loose (areolar) or dense categories depending on the arrangement of the protein fibres
- reticular connective tissue has fine fibres of reticulin which form a fine supporting meshwork
- adipose connective tissue in which adipocytes (fat) cells are predominant.

Connective tissue proper

Loose areolar connective tissue

Loose areolar connective tissue occupies spaces that no other organs or tissues occupy: it is packing material. It underlies the skin (the hypodermis), surrounds

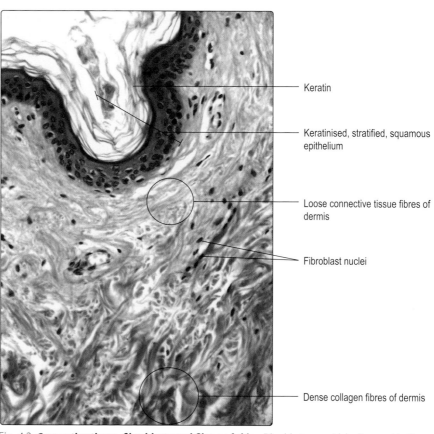

Fig. 4.2 **Connective tissue, fibroblasts and fibres of skin.** Fibroblasts are widely dispersed in the extracellular matrix of the dermis. In the deeper region, densely packed collagen fibres are predominant. Medium magnification.

Labels in figure:
- Keratin
- Keratinised, stratified, squamous epithelium
- Loose connective tissue fibres of dermis
- Fibroblast nuclei
- Dense collagen fibres of dermis

Clinical notes

Vitamin C deficiency Vitamin C is essential for the synthesis of normal collagen. Normally, collagen molecules are replaced several months after they are formed by new collagen. If vitamin C is absent from the diet for prolonged periods the condition known as scurvy develops and the new collagen that replaces the old is abnormal. Collagen attaches teeth to the sockets in jaw bones; in extremely severe cases of scurvy, the teeth drop out of the sockets because the new collagen is defective.

Marfan syndrome In this condition a genetic mutation results in the abnormal function of elastin fibres in the body. Many regions are affected but, in particular, the loss of the normal elastin component in the wall of the aorta (the main blood vessel from the heart supplying the body) can be serious as the wall may rupture; this is usually fatal.

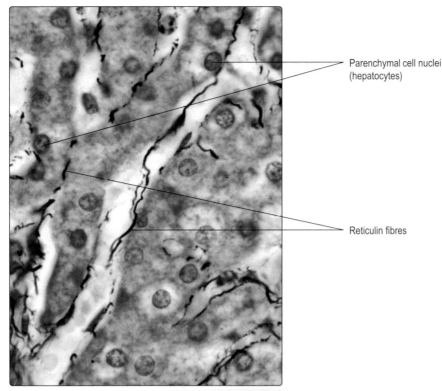

Fig. 4.3 **Reticulin fibres in liver.** Reticulin fibres appear as thin, dark brown strands. They provide support for liver parenchymal epithelial cells (hepatocytes). Special stain. High magnification.

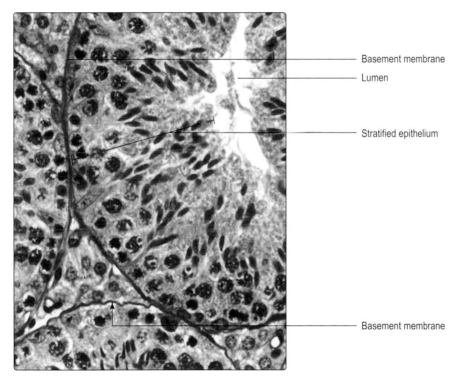

Fig. 4.4 **Basement membrane supporting a stratified epithelium in the testis.** This epithelium lines tubules and is attached to a basement membrane which appears magenta as its content of glycoproteins has been stained. Special stain. High magnification.

port of gases and other molecules between blood vessels and surrounding cells and is a region where various cell types such as the cells of the immune system (Chapter 8) can interact. Transient cell types such as white blood cells may also be present in areolar tissue. Loose connective tissue may respond to trauma or infection by becoming oedematous and infiltrated by increased numbers of white blood cells and other immune-related cells (signs of inflammation).

Loose connective tissue is characterised by abundant amounts of ground substance, and by fibroblasts which are usually widely spaced and may appear to have little or no cytoplasm. In histological sections ground substance may appear as empty spaces since many components may have been extracted during the processing of the tissue. Also present in loose connective tissue are varying proportions of collagen and elastin which appear as pink strands in routine H&E preparations (Figs 4.1 and 4.2). Some components of connective tissue can be more readily revealed by various special staining techniques (Figs 4.6 and 4.7).

Dense connective tissue

Dense connective tissue may be classified as regular or irregular with regard to the arrangement of the fibres. The former is arranged as bundles of similarly oriented, densely packed collagen fibres which resist tensile forces, such as those applied to tendons (Fig. 4.8) and ligaments. The predominant cell type is the fibroblast. However, given the tight packing of the collagen fibres, there is relatively little space for extracellular matrix or transient cells. Dense, irregular connective tissue also has densely packed collagen fibres, but they are arranged irregularly and resist tensile forces from many directions. Again, the predominant cell type is the fibroblast and there is little space for extracellular material or transient cells. A typical site for this type of connective tissue is the deep region of the dermis of the skin (Fig. 4.2).

Reticular connective tissue

The fine collagen fibres of reticulin act as a delicate framework for the parenchymal cells of several organs, e.g. the liver (Fig. 4.3) and endocrine glands (Fig. 4.7), where minimal impedance to the transport of large molecules is important. Reticulin also provides a support network for immune cells in the

delicate organs and skeletal muscles, and acts as filler around blood vessels and nerves. Loose connective tissue physically connects many parts of the body, e.g. it binds together the constituents of the walls of the gastrointestinal, respiratory, urinary and reproductive tracts. It is also present in the delicate membranes attaching organs or tubes to other structures, e.g. the membranes of the gut (Fig. 4.6). In addition to its 'connective' role, areolar tissue also acts as a medium for the trans-

spleen, bone marrow and lymph nodes (Chapter 8).

Adipose connective tissue

There are two types of adipose tissue: white adipose and brown adipose tissue. White adipose tissue is the most prominent type in adults. It is also known as unilocular fat as each cell contains one fat droplet which occupies most of the cell. In brown fat, known as multilocular fat, the constituent cells store the fat as multiple droplets. Both types of adipose tissue have many blood vessels. White adipose tissue contains connective tissue fibres forming septa that break the tissue up into lobules (Fig. 4.1). This type of adipose tissue is found under the skin (subcutaneously), and it may be extensive in particular regions of the body. Brown fat is a reddish brown colour in life and its cells contain abundant mitochondria. The latter are related to its principal function, which is to release energy from the fat its cells contain. Much of this energy is heat and it aids temperature regulation in neonates. Brown fat is found in particular locations in the body; it is most evident in infants, although it is also found in the neck region of adults.

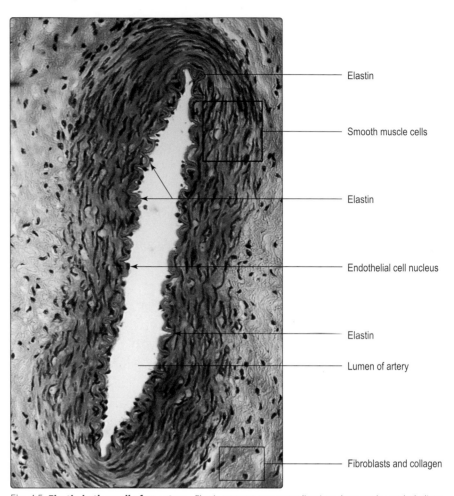

Elastin
Smooth muscle cells
Elastin
Endothelial cell nucleus
Elastin
Lumen of artery
Fibroblasts and collagen

Fig. 4.5 **Elastin in the wall of an artery.** Elastin appears as a wavy line just deep to the endothelium lining the lumen of this artery. The elastin has recoiled, hence the wavy line. The nuclei of the endothelial cells bulge into the lumen. Layers of muscle cells, known as smooth muscle, form part of the wall. Medium magnification.

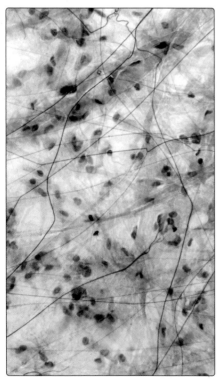

Fig. 4.6 **A whole (not sectioned) thin membrane.** Some irregularly distributed protein fibres stain green and vary in thickness. Other thin fibres (reticulin) stain dark brown. Nuclei of connective tissue and epithelial cells stain purple. Special stain. High magnification.

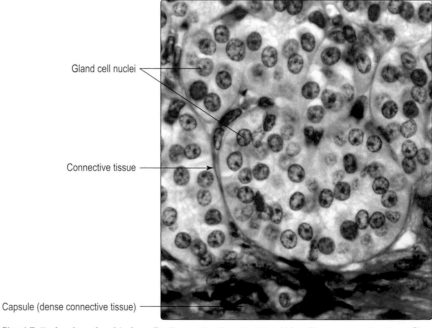

Gland cell nuclei
Connective tissue
Capsule (dense connective tissue)

Fig. 4.7 **Endocrine gland (adrenal).** Connective tissue is stained blue. Dense connective tissue fibres surround the gland as a capsule and fine connective tissue fibres support the gland cells. Special stain. High magnification.

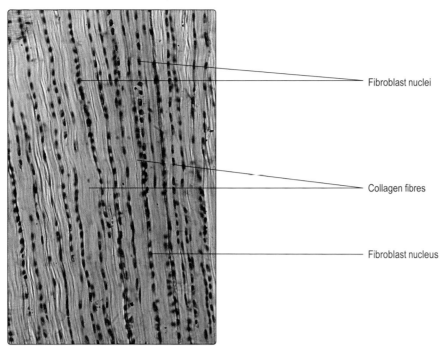

Fibroblast nuclei

Collagen fibres

Fibroblast nucleus

Fig. 4.8 **Dense regular connective tissue of a tendon.** The collagen fibres are distributed in parallel arrays and nuclei of fibroblasts appear as dark dots in rows between the fibres. Medium magnification.

Summary

Connective tissue:

- consists of connective tissue cells in extracellular matrix (ECM)
  - the cells in many connective tissues are widely spaced
  - blood and bone and cartilage are specialised connective tissues.

Cells in connective tissue include:

- fibroblasts which synthesise the protein fibres and other large molecules in the ECM
- mast cells which synthesise, store and secrete molecules that affect the permeability of blood vessels
- macrophages which phagocytose and digest cell debris and microorganisms, and aid immune responses
- white blood cells which migrate through the ECM and may remain localised as part of the immune response
- adipocytes which store lipids.

Extracellular matrix consists of:

- ground substance containing
  - water, salts, dissolved gases and small molecules
  - large molecules, e.g. glycoproteins, proteoglycans and glycosoaminoglycans which affect the viscosity and function of the ECM
  - molecules to which cells involved in immune responses adhere
- protein fibres
  - collagen types I and II provide strength, e.g. in skin
  - collagen type III (also known as reticulin) provides delicate meshworks which support other cells, e.g. in the liver
  - collagen type IV forms basement membranes which support many epithelial cells
  - elastin fibres which are able to stretch and recoil.

Categories of connective tissues (other than bone, cartilage and blood) are:

- proper connective tissue
  - loose connective tissue connects structures
  - dense connective tissue has little ECM
- reticulin connective tissue
- adipose connective tissue.

Chapter 5
Primary tissues 3: muscle tissue

Muscle tissue consists of cells which are able to contract. The fundamental characteristic of each muscle cell is that it has contractile proteins (mainly the myofilaments actin and myosin) in its cytoplasm. The force generated by the contraction of these proteins is transmitted via connective tissue to other structures. Contraction of muscles attached (by connective tissue) to bones will either move the bones at their joints or stabilise the bones and joints by resisting forces produced by other contracting muscles and by gravity. Contraction of muscles in the walls of various structures in the body may increase the pressure within these structures and thus perform vital functions, e.g. heart muscle contraction ensures blood flows away from the heart and muscle in the walls of gut tubes ensures the gut contents pass from mouth to anus.

Specific terms have been introduced to identify particular parts of muscle cells (which are also known as muscle fibres). The muscle cell membrane is known as the sarcolemma, the cytoplasm as the sarcoplasm and the smooth endoplasmic reticulum as the sarcoplasmic reticulum.

Types of muscle tissue

There are three types of muscle tissue classified by location and the arrangement of the contractile myofilaments in the muscle cells:

- *skeletal* muscle contraction is involved, mainly, in moving the skeleton
- *cardiac* muscle contraction moves blood through the heart
- *smooth* muscle in the walls of many tubes and hollow organs (e.g. in some blood vessels and the urinary bladder) controls the flow of substances along or out of such structures.

Skeletal and cardiac muscle cells are referred to as striped or striated muscle as the contractile myofilaments are arranged in a repeating pattern in the sarcoplasm and this is manifested as transverse dark and light striations across the length of the muscle cells (Figs 5.1A,B and 5.2). The precise arrangement of the contractile myofilaments are revealed only by using an electron microscope (see below). Although smooth muscle cells contain actin and myosin myofilaments, they are not arranged in a regular pattern and smooth muscle cells do not display striations (Fig. 5.1C).

Other cell types with the ability to contract have also been detected using techniques which identify contractile proteins in their cytoplasm. These types include:

- *myoepithelial cells*, which surround acini and ducts of some exocrine glands; their contraction aids the expulsion of secretions
- *myofibroblasts*, which occur in many regions of connective tissue; they aid repair by secreting collagen and undergoing contraction during scar formation
- *pericytes*, which surround capillaries; after injury they undergo mitosis and replace damaged fibroblasts and smooth muscle cells.

Muscle cells and connective tissue

Confusingly, muscle cells are also referred to as muscle fibres, probably because some are long, thin structures which measure several centimetres in length. (In contrast, connective tissue

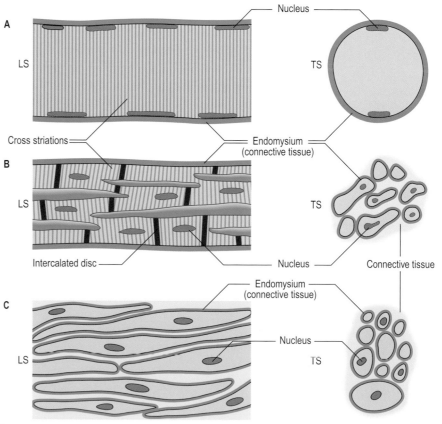

Fig. 5.1 **The longitudinal (LS) and transverse (TS) appearance of (A) skeletal, (B) cardiac and (C) smooth muscle as revealed by light microscopy.**

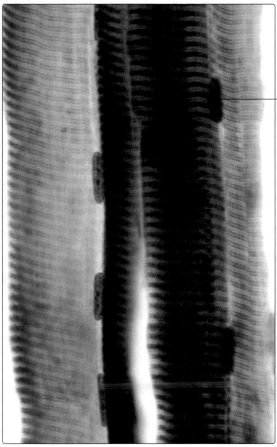

Skeletal muscle cell nucleus

Fig. 5.2 **Skeletal muscle cells sectioned along their length.** Light and dark transverse striations occur along the length of muscle cells and are due to the regularity of the arrangement of the myofibrils and myofilaments (actin and myosin) in the sarcoplasm. (The myofibrils and myofilaments themselves are not revealed by light microscopy.) Special stain. Very high power.

fibres, although long and thin, are protein molecules, not cells.)

The connective tissue associated with muscle cells consists of three covering layers (Figs 5.1 and 5.3). Each muscle cell is covered by, and bound to, fine connective tissue fibres which form an external (basal) lamina known as an endomysium. Several muscle cells are held together as bundles by connective tissue fibres known as the perimysium. The connective tissue covering a muscle itself, e.g. the biceps brachii, is called the epimysium; this layer is also known as deep fascia.

Contraction of a muscle, such as biceps brachii, involves the contractile proteins in individual muscle cells moving and shortening their overall length. This movement generates a force of contraction and it is transmitted to the sarcolemma and the external lamina. The laminae around adjacent muscle cells are connected to each other and to the other layers of connective tissue. In this way the force of muscle cell contraction is transmitted to all the connective tissue layers. Such contractile forces from muscle cells, applied to connective

tissue fibres, is then transferred to other structures such as bone e.g. the humerus or soft tissue, e.g. the eyeball.

It is important to appreciate that when muscles stop contracting they passively relax and the contractile proteins resume their original position but this does not exert a force. Muscles can only contract (pull), never push!

Skeletal muscle

As its name suggests this type of muscle is associated with the skeletal system, and it is responsible for movements of bones and joints. Skeletal muscle is also known as voluntary muscle as its contraction is usually under conscious control via its nerve supply. Skeletal muscle gives characteristic form to the body's contour (along with adipose tissue). Although gross anatomy is beyond the scope of this book, it is important to appreciate that the attachment sites of a skeletal muscle to the skeleton, and the position of the muscle in relation to a joint, will determine the line of pull of the muscle and the type of movement that occurs at the joint as the muscle contracts.

Skeletal muscle cells are multinucleate, long and cylindrical in shape. They form by fusion of several cells (myoblasts) during development in utero. The nuclei of skeletal muscle cells are at the periphery of the sarcoplasm (Figs 5.1A and 5.2), a feature which allows them to be distinguished from other types of muscle cell. The contractile myofilaments (actin and myosin) within muscle cells are arranged as bundles (myofibrils) with their long axes along the length of the cells (Fig. 5.3) and each cell contains hundreds of myofibrils. The contractile proteins in the myofibrils overlap each other (Fig. 5.4A) and form a functional unit (a sarcomere). Aligned in this way the myofibrils refract light differently, hence the striped appearance (Fig. 5.2). The dark bands are known as A bands and the I bands are light.

In histological sections of skeletal muscle cells which have been sectioned along their length, transverse striations, reflecting the arrangement of the contractile proteins, are apparent (Fig. 5.2). If skeletal muscle cells are not sectioned along their length the striations are not apparent, but it is possible to recognise the type of muscle cell by the peripheral position of the nuclei (Figs 5.1A and 5.5). Numerous blood capillaries (Fig. 5.6) can be demonstrated in the connective tissue layers around muscle cells. The capillaries ensure a good blood supply, which provides the oxygen and nutrients necessary for muscle contraction.

Many skeletal muscles are anchored to bone by tendons (Chapter 4). The collagen fibres covering the muscle cells are continuous with the collagen of the tendon. In turn, bundles of collagen, known as Sharpey's fibres, pass into the bone and anchor the tendon. Tendons take on a variety of forms, such that the attachment may be focal or broad. In some muscles the connective tissue surrounding the muscle cells attaches to a collagen (fascial) layer (Fig. 5.7), rather than to bone.

Variation occurs in the size of muscle cells, the number of mitochondria they contain and the enzymes present, as well as their content of myoglobin. Myoglobin, an oxygen-carrying protein, resembles haemoglobin and gives muscle a reddish colour. Such red muscle cells are predominant in muscles in which sustained contraction is required, e.g. to maintain posture. In contrast, in muscles where fast contraction and spurts of activity occur myoglobin is sparse and the muscles appear whitish to the naked eye.

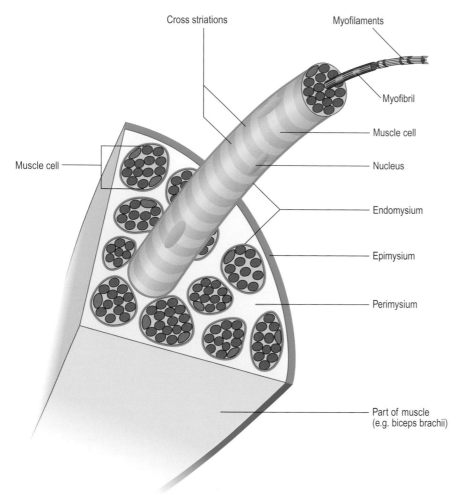

Cross striations · Myofilaments · Myofibril · Muscle cell · Nucleus · Endomysium · Epimysium · Perimysium · Muscle cell · Part of muscle (e.g. biceps brachii)

Fig. 5.3 **The three connective tissue layers covering muscle cells in part of a muscle.** Myofilaments in one myofibril of a muscle cell are shown.

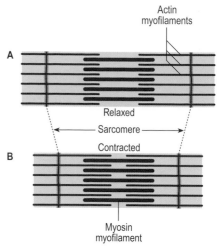

Actin myofilaments · A · Relaxed · Sarcomere · Contracted · B · Myosin myofilament

Fig. 5.4 **The arrangement of actin and myosin myofilaments in a sarcomere in the relaxed (A) and the contracted (B) state.**

Ultrastructure of skeletal muscle and contraction

Contractile proteins occupy much of the sarcoplasm of muscle cells, and the thick myosin and thin actin myofilaments can be identified in cells sectioned longitudinally and transversely (Figs 5.8 and 5.9 respectively). Numerous mitochondria (Fig. 5.9) are present in muscle cells and myoglobin and glycogen may also be present; all aid in providing energy for contraction. An extensive membranous meshwork connecting the sarcolemma and the sarcoplasmic reticulum (the t tubule system) is present (Fig. 5.9). This meshwork has a role in moving calcium ions into the sarcoplasm, which is a process that is an essential trigger for muscle contraction.

The functional unit of the skeletal muscle cell is known as a sarcomere (Fig. 5.4) and it consists of thin (actin) and thick (myosin) myofilaments and other proteins which anchor them in parallel arrays and to the sarcolemma. Contraction involves the parallel actin and myosin proteins sliding along each other (Fig. 5.4), thus shortening the cell overall. This is known as the sliding filament mechanism of contraction and is an energy-dependent process.

Cardiac muscle

This type of muscle, like skeletal muscle, appears striated (Figs 5.1B and 5.10) owing to the arrangement of the actin and myosin proteins in the sarcoplasm. Unlike skeletal muscle, cardiac muscle contraction is not under conscious control. Cardiac muscle cells are cylindrical and much shorter than skeletal muscle cells. Each cardiac muscle cell has a single, centrally placed nucleus

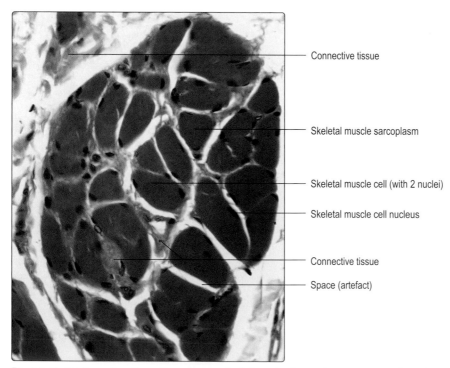

Connective tissue · Skeletal muscle sarcoplasm · Skeletal muscle cell (with 2 nuclei) · Skeletal muscle cell nucleus · Connective tissue · Space (artefact)

Fig. 5.5 **Skeletal muscle cells sectioned across their length.** Connective tissue surrounds each muscle cell and groups of muscle cells. Some spaces are artefacts due to shrinkage during preparation of the section. High magnification.

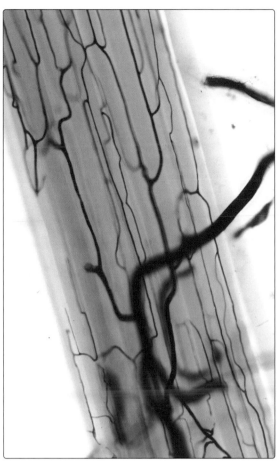

Fig. 5.6 **Skeletal muscle cells (yellow) sectioned along their length showing blood vessels (red).** A rich network of small blood vessels passes, in connective tissue, along the length of the muscle cells. (No details of the muscle cell structure or connective tissue are displayed.) Special stain. Medium magnification.

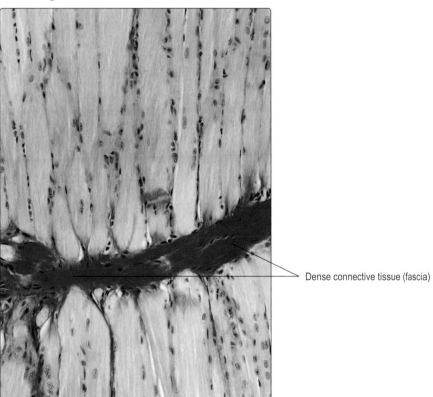

Dense connective tissue (fascia)

Fig. 5.7 **Skeletal muscle cells (yellow) from tongue.** The skeletal muscle cells are sectioned along their length and display their peripheral nuclei. Connective tissue (stained red) surrounds each muscle cell and provides a dense fascial layer of collagen to which the muscle cells are attached. Forces from contraction of the muscle cells are transferred to the connective tissue and change the shape of the tongue. Special stain. Low magnification.

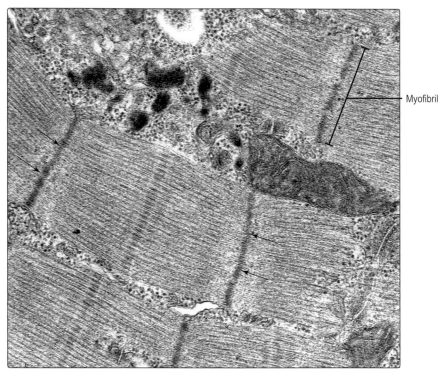

Fig. 5.8 **Electron micrograph of part of the sarcoplasm of a skeletal muscle cell sectioned along its length.** The length of a sarcomere in a myofibril is indicated by arrows. Thick (myosin) and thin (actin) myofilaments can be seen in parallel linear arrays in the sarcomere (and in other regions of the myofibrils shown) as thick (myosin) and thinner (actin) lines. High magnification.

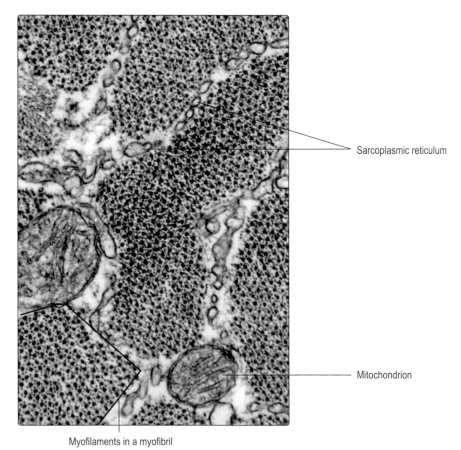

Fig. 5.9 **Electron micrograph of part of the sarcoplasm of a skeletal muscle cell sectioned across its length.** Myosin (thick) and actin (thin) myofilaments can be seen sectioned across their length in several myofibrils as dark dots (myosin) and smaller, paler dots (actin). Very high magnification.

and some cells branch (Fig. 5.1B). Specialised cell junctions (Chapter 2) link cardiac muscle cells end to end and these regions, called intercalated discs, are visible in histological sections (Fig. 5.10). Desmosomes and zonulae adherens anchor the muscle cells together at intercalated discs. In addition, there are gap junctions at these discs which ensure the excitation stimulating contraction spreads rapidly between muscle cells and results in their synchronised contraction. The mechanism of contraction is similar to that of skeletal muscle. The connective tissue associated with cardiac muscle (Fig. 5.10) is arranged in layers similar to those of skeletal muscle and it transmits the forces of the muscle contraction. The arrangement of connective tissue fibres forms a fibrous 'skeleton' for the heart. This arrangement helps to ensure that the contraction of heart muscle cells constricts the chambers of the heart in synchrony and it also anchors the heart valves and aids their function (Chapter 10).

Smooth muscle

Smooth muscle cells are fusiform in shape and tapered at each end with a centrally placed nucleus (Fig. 5.1C). Smooth muscle cells are usually grouped together and form sheets or bundles, and their appearance in histological sections depends on the angle at which they are sectioned (Figs 5.1C and 5.11) and their state of contraction (Fig. 5.12). Contraction of smooth muscle cells is not under conscious control and they are described as involuntary muscle cells. The contractile proteins in smooth muscle cells are arranged irregularly and some are linked with adherens-type junctions at intervals on the inner surface of the cell membrane. Each muscle cell is attached to an external lamina of connective tissue (endomysium) (Fig. 5.1C) and muscle cells are bundled together by layers of connective tissue (Fig. 5.11). Between some muscle cells the external lamina is incomplete and gap junctions link adjacent smooth muscle cells. The presence of gap junctions aids the spread of the excitatory stimulus for contraction and helps groups of cells to contract as a single unit. When smooth muscle cells contract they take on a corkscrew-like shape, which may be apparent as a change in shape of the nucleus (Fig. 5.12), and the force is transmitted via their external laminae to other surrounding connective tissue.

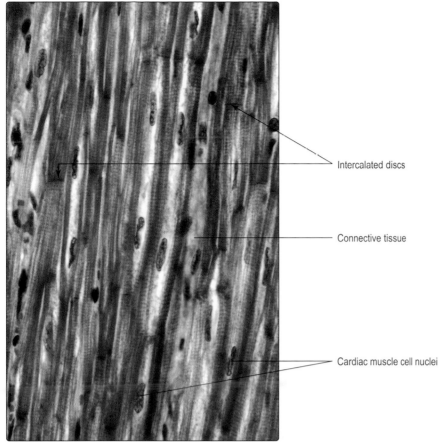

Fig. 5.10 **Cardiac muscle cells sectioned along their length and associated connective tissue (blue/green).** Special stain. Medium magnification.

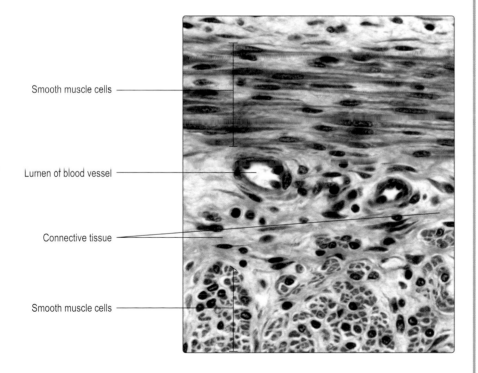

Fig. 5.11 **Bundles of smooth muscle cells sectioned along their length (upper region) and across their length (lower region).** Many of the smooth muscle cells sectioned across their length do not appear to have nuclei as the section has passed though a region of cytoplasm away from the nucleus. The nucleus and cytoplasm of smooth muscle cells sectioned longitudinally appear elongated as the long axis of each cell is in the plane of the section. Connective tissue (green) surrounds and separates the muscle cells and bundles, and two small blood vessels. Special stain. Medium magnification.

Muscle contraction and nerve supply

Skeletal muscle contraction is dependent on its nerve supply. Indeed, if the nerves supplying skeletal muscles are severed the muscle cells do not contract and they waste away (atrophy). Cardiac and smooth muscle cells have an intrinsic ability to contract in the absence of nerve supply. However, they are supplied by nerves which control their activity but they are not normally under conscious control. Further details of the nerve supply to muscles is given in Chapter 6.

> *Clinical note*
> **Muscle hypertrophy, hyperplasia and repair** Adult skeletal muscle is able to undergo hypertrophy: the muscle cells become larger as they respond to exercise by forming more contractile proteins. Although skeletal muscle cells are not able to undergo mitosis, if very minor damage occurs some repair may occur. This is due to a minor population of undifferentiated cells (known as satellite cells) in skeletal muscle which can differentiate into skeletal muscle cells.
>
> Cardiac muscle cells can also increase in volume by hypertrophy, and this can occur in response to high blood pressure (hypertension). In contrast to skeletal muscle, there are no stem cells in cardiac muscle and so there is no replacement of dead cardiac muscle cells. After a heart attack (myocardial infarction), cardiac muscle cells die because of loss of their blood supply and they are not replaced. Fibroblasts in the connective tissue of the heart proliferate and secrete collagen and a fibrous scar takes the place of the dead muscle cells. The scar may alter the contraction of the normal heart muscle with harmful consequences.
>
> Smooth muscle cells can undergo hypertrophy (increase in cell size) and hyperplasia (increase in cell number). These processes are particularly important in ensuring uterine muscle is able to function during pregnancy and childbirth.

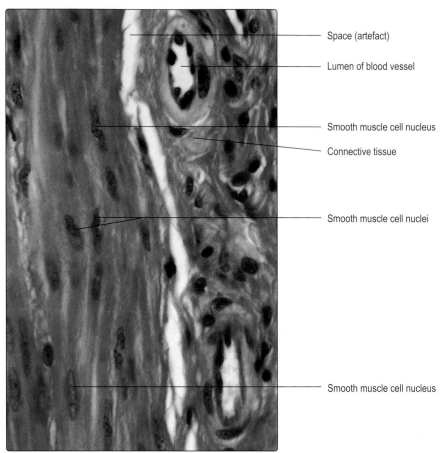

Space (artefact)

Lumen of blood vessel

Smooth muscle cell nucleus

Connective tissue

Smooth muscle cell nuclei

Smooth muscle cell nucleus

Fig. 5.12 **Smooth muscle cells sectioned along their length.** Some nuclei of smooth muscle cells appear normal (fusiform) in shape; others appear kinked, which is typical of smooth muscle cells fixed in a state of contraction. Some spaces are artefacts due to shrinkage during processing. Other spaces are the lumina of blood vessels lined by endothelial cells. High magnification.

Summary

Muscle tissue
- Muscle tissue comprises three main types of muscle cell:
  - skeletal, cardiac and smooth.
- Myoepithelial cells, myofibroblasts and pericytes also have the ability to contract.
- Intracytoplasmic proteins (mainly the myofilaments actin and myosin) in muscle cells (and the above cell types) are responsible for contraction.
- Connective tissue adjacent to muscle cells transmits the force of contraction to other structures.

Skeletal muscle
- Cells are multinucleate and nuclei are adjacent to the sarcolemma (muscle cell membrane).
- Cells are long, cylindrical and display transverse striations reflecting the linear arrangement of the myofilaments in the sarcoplasm (cytoplasm).
- Contraction moves bones at joints and/or stabilises joints.
- Contraction is (mostly) under conscious control via the nerve supply.

Cardiac muscle
- Cells are cylindrical, relatively short, and have a single, centrally placed nucleus.
- Cells display transverse striations corresponding to the linear arrangement of myofilaments.
- Cells have intercalated discs showing the end-to-end connection of these cells.
- Contraction is under the (unconscious) control of nerves.
- Contractions, transmitted to connective tissue in the heart, move blood through the heart in a synchronised manner.

Smooth muscle
- Cells are fusiform in shape and a nucleus is in the centre of each cell.
- Cells have few randomly arranged myofilaments.
- Cells occur in bundles or layers around many tubes.
- Contraction is under (unconscious) control of nerves.

Chapter 6
Primary tissues 4: nerve tissue

Nerve tissue comprises neurons (nerve cells) and a range of cells that support the neurons, e.g. glial and satellite cells. Nerve tissue is involved in carrying rapid, specific communications between various parts of the body. Neurons gather information, process it and transmit signals to other neurons or other cell types (e.g. muscle and gland cells). The transmitted signals affect the function of the recipient cells.

Nerve tissue and the nervous system

The nervous system has two structural components. Nerve tissue located in the brain and spinal cord is the major component of the central nervous system (CNS). Other primary tissues are present in the CNS though they are sparse, e.g. connective tissue provides some support. The peripheral nervous system (PNS) comprises nerve tissue which is not in the CNS, e.g. cranial and spinal nerves and their branches, and autonomic nerves (see below). Connective tissue also has a supporting role in the PNS.

The nervous system has two functional components, somatic and autonomic. The somatic nervous system involves the detection of sensations and the control of skeletal muscle contraction. Some sensations are not consciously perceived, such as a change in tension in a tendon, though the change detected can cause a response, such as contraction of skeletal muscle(s). The functions of the autonomic nervous system (ANS) involve the control of contraction of smooth and cardiac muscle cells and the secretory activity of some gland cells. The ANS, in general, is not under conscious control. However, an important exception is that the autonomic nerves involved in controlling the smooth muscle cells in the wall of the urinary bladder are normally under conscious control by the age of 2–3 years.

Neurons

Neurons are derived from the ectoderm germ layer of the embryo (see Mitchell B, Sharma R. *Embryology: An Illustrated Colour Text.* Elsevier: 2004). Most neurons have a large mass of cytoplasm and large nucleus forming the body of the cell (the perikaryon) and a variable number of cytoplasmic processes (Fig. 6.1). Perikarya may measure up to 150 μm in diameter, which is about 20 times larger than a red blood cell. The cytoplasmic processes are of two forms, dendrites and axons. Most neurons have several short dendrites that receive signals which they then pass to their own cell body. In general, each neuron has a long, single axon which takes signals away from the perikaryon either to other neurons or to other cell types, e.g. muscle cells. Axons may be up to about a metre in length in humans, i.e. the length from the lower regions of the spinal cord to the foot.

In routine H&E stained sections, neuronal nuclei have large, palely stained areas (Fig. 6.2). Such areas represent uncoiled euchromatin, the hallmark of DNA transcription and a prerequisite for protein synthesis. The cytoplasm in neuronal cell bodies often appears granular, especially if special stains have been used (Fig. 6.3). The granules are referred to as Nissl granules and they are due to large accumulations of rough endoplasmic reticulum (RER), which are involved in the synthesis of various proteins. Some of these proteins provide the structural tubules and filaments in axons and dendrites. Others are enzymes involved in producing molecules which aid the transmission of signals.

Neurons vary in shape and size, and according to function and location. The complexity of their cytoplasmic processes is vast and revealed by special stains (Fig. 6.4).

- *Variation in shape.* Neurons are classified as multipolar (Fig. 6.1), bipolar or pseudounipolar (Fig. 6.5). The polarity is related to the number of cytoplasmic processes projecting from the perikaryon. Many neurons are multipolar and, typically, one axon and many dendrites extend from the perikaryon (Fig. 6.1). Some neurons in the brain and ventral regions (horns) of the spinal cord are multipolar. Bipolar neurons are present in organs of the special senses (e.g. the eye) and they have two cytoplasmic processes, one an

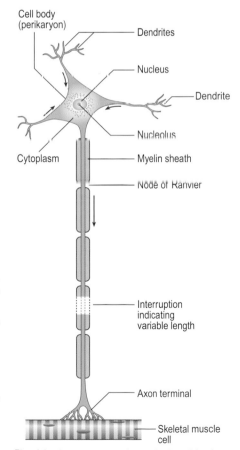

Fig. 6.1 **The structure of a typical multipolar neuron (a motor neuron with its axon ensheathed in myelin).** Arrows indicate the direction of travel of the nerve impulse.

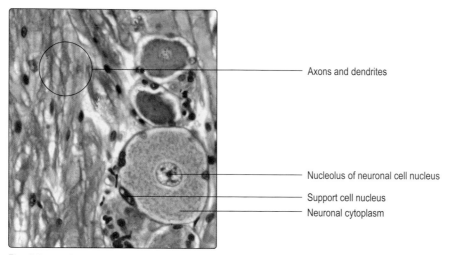

Fig. 6.2 **Ganglion.** A neuronal cell body (perikaryon) with palely stained nucleus and densely stained nucleolus and extensive cytoplasm. The cytoplasm of axons and dendrites cannot be distinguished: both appear as pink strands. High magnification.

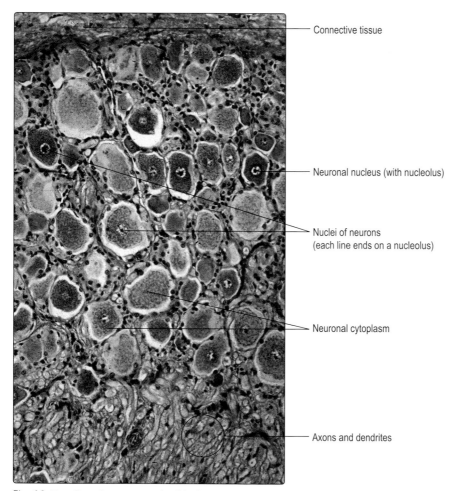

Fig. 6.3 **Ganglion.** Some neuronal cell bodies appear to lack a nucleus; this is because a section 5 μm thick through neuronal cell bodies which may be 150 μm in diameter could miss the nucleus. Connective tissue (blue) surrounds and is within the ganglion. Special stain. Medium magnification.

axon and one a dendrite. Pseudounipolar neurons possess one process, though it bifurcates and one branch receives signals and the other branch transmits them away from the cell body. Examples of pseudounipolar neurons are those that transmit sensory information from the skin.

■ *Variation in function.* All neurons respond to stimuli by transmitting signals along their axons, away from their cell body. The signals are in the form of nerve (electrical) impulses which move rapidly along the axon. As the nerve impulses reach the terminal part of the axon the signal is passed on by various molecules (neurotransmitters) released from the axon. The neurotransmitters stimulate a response in the target cell. If the target cell is another neuron the signal continues as a nerve impulse. If the target cell is a muscle cell, the neurotransmitter stimulates the muscle cell membrane and this results in the muscle cell undergoing contraction.

The rate at which nerve impulses are transmitted along axons varies. In general, the wider the diameter of an axon, the faster the nerve impulse travels. The speed of transmission of nerve impulses is also higher in axons that are sheathed in myelin (Fig. 6.1). Myelin is a lipid bilayer arranged as concentric, multiple layers around some axons (Figs 6.6A, 6.7 and 6.8). The layers are formed from the cell membranes of Schwann cells in the PNS and, in the CNS, from the cell membranes of certain glial cells (oligodendrocytes). In places, the myelin sheaths around axons are not layered and these regions are described as nodes of Ranvier (Figs 6.1 and 6.9). The nodes are the interface between two adjacent myelin-producing cells and they are important in ensuring a relatively rapid rate of transmission of the nerve impulse. Other axons are not ensheathed in myelin, but several axons are indented into the cytoplasm of one myelin-producing Schwann cell (Fig. 6.6B). Transmission of impulses along these non-myelinated axons is relatively slow.

■ *Variation in location.* Afferent neurons carry sensory signals to the CNS and efferent neurons carry signals away from the CNS to

Neuronal cytoplasmic process

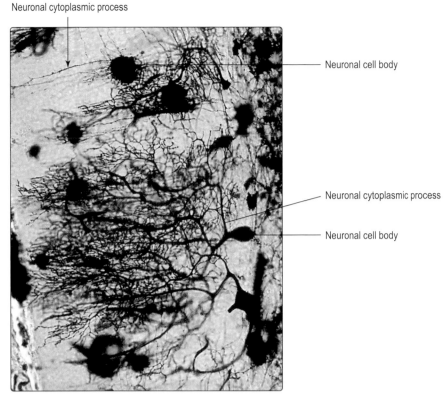

Neuronal cell body

Neuronal cytoplasmic process

Neuronal cell body

Fig. 6.4 **Neurons in brain.** Perikarya and numerous cytoplasmic processes show some of the variation and complexity of their connections. Special stain. Medium magnification.

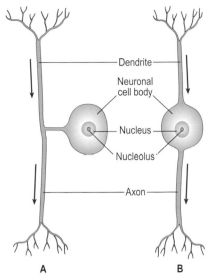

Dendrite

Neuronal cell body

Nucleus

Nucleolus

Axon

A

B

Fig. 6.5 **The structure of (A) a pseudounipolar and (B) a bipolar neuron.** Arrows indicate the direction of travel of the nerve impulse.

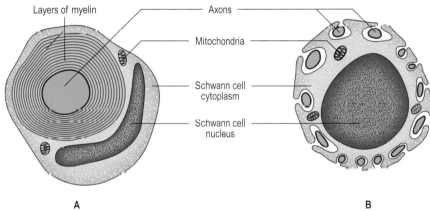

Layers of myelin

Axons

Mitochondria

Schwann cell cytoplasm

Schwann cell nucleus

A

B

Fig. 6.6 **The relationship of a Schwann cell and myelin in a transverse section of (A) a myelinated axon and (B) non-myelinated axons.**

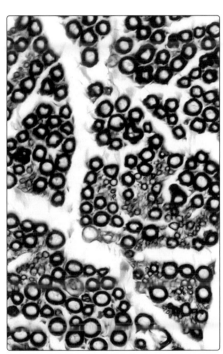

Fig. 6.7 **Peripheral nerve (with cytoplasmic processes of many neurons) sectioned across its length.** The lipids in Schwann cell membranes which form myelin sheaths are shown as black circles. The axons which occupy the centre of the circles are not stained. Special stain. High magnification.

various cells, e.g. muscle and gland cells. Afferent nerves enter the spinal cord by dorsal roots and efferent nerves leave by ventral roots (Fig. 6.10). Some afferent neurons communicate directly in the CNS with efferent neurons and form a two-neuron reflex arc (pathway) (Fig. 6.10A). Others transmit information to interneurons in the spinal cord which in turn communicate with efferent neurons in a three-neuron arc (Fig. 6.10B). In both types of reflex arc other neurons transmit impulses to the brain.

Afferent (sensory) neurons provide a variety of information. Some afferent neurons have specialised structures known as sensory receptors (Fig. 6.11) at the peripheral end of a cytoplasmic process; others end as 'free nerve endings'. Sensory receptors in, for example, the skin detect sensations, and nerve impulses are transmitted to the CNS. Sensory receptors in skin can provide impulses that are perceived as pain, touch (differentiating type and pressure) and temperature. Signals from sensory receptors in some organs may be perceived as changes in pressure or amount of stretch. Other sensory receptors convey information which is not perceived consciously, e.g. changes in blood pressure, but the body responds to the changes detected. Highly specialised sensory neurons are present in the organs involved in sight, hearing, smell and taste; for information about these, a more detailed histology book should be consulted.

Efferent neurons transmit impulses away from the CNS and

affect the function of other neurons and other cells, e.g. gland and muscle cells (efferent neurons which stimulate muscle contraction are known as motor neurons (Fig. 6.1)). There are two categories of efferent neuron:

- *Somatic efferent neurons.* These stimulate skeletal muscle contraction and may involve a series of nerve impulses originating in the brain after conscious thought. Skeletal muscle contraction may also occur as a reflex response, e.g. to a painful stimulus. The sensory information passes in a reflex arc through the spinal cord (Fig. 6.10) and directly (or via an interneuron) to one or more efferent motor neurons which stimulate muscle contraction. This reflex pathway does not involve the brain but neurons relay the pain sensations rapidly to the brain and then the pain is perceived.
- *Autonomic efferent neurons.* These control smooth muscle contraction, e.g. smooth muscle in the walls of blood vessels and the walls of the digestive, respiratory, reproductive and urinary tracts. Autonomic efferent nerves also control the contraction of cardiac muscle cells and gland cell secretion, e.g. by salivary and sweat glands.

Synapses

Synapses are specialised cell junctions between neurons or between neurons and other cell types, e.g. muscle cells. The commonest form of synapse is the axo-dendritic synapse formed between the axon of a neuron and the dendrite(s) of another neuron.

All synapses have similar characteristics (Fig. 6.12). In axo-dendritic synapses the membrane of the terminal part of the axon of the presynaptic cell lies in close apposition to the membrane of a dendrite of the postsynaptic cell. The space between the two cells is known as the synaptic cleft. The neuron transmitting the nerve impulse to a synapse has a presynaptic axonal swelling in which numerous cellular organelles and synaptic vesicles are present. The synaptic vesicles are small membrane-bound structures containing neurotransmitter molecules. The morphology of synaptic vesicles is related to their content. The main neurotransmitters include acetyl-

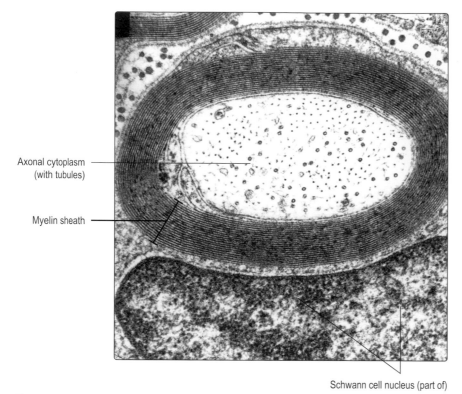

Fig. 6.8 **Electron micrograph of a transverse section of an axon and surrounding myelin sheath.** Very high magnification.

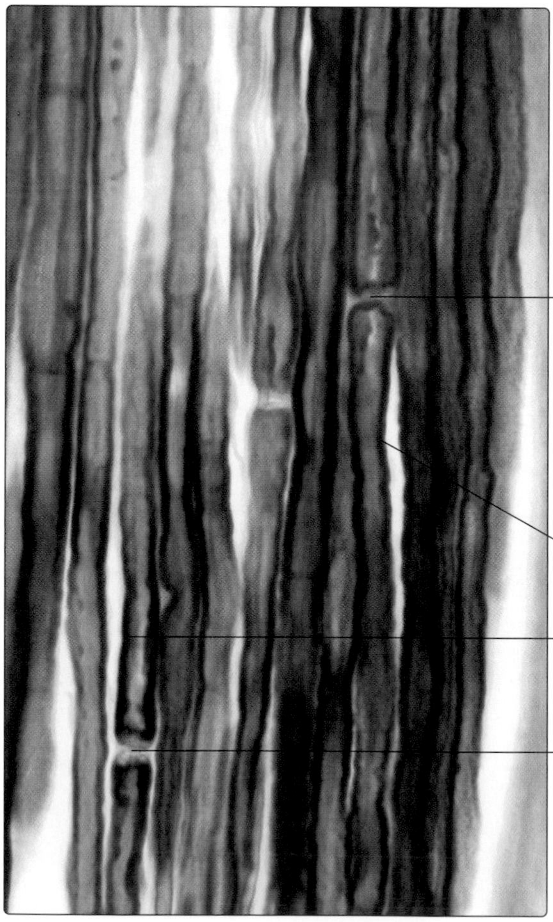

Fig. 6.9 **Cytoplasmic processes (axons) of neurons sectioned along their length.** Special stain. Very high magnification.

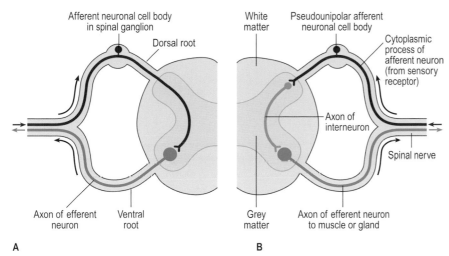

Fig. 6.10 **The spinal cord (sectioned transversely) showing grey and white matter.** Arrows show the routes taken by sensory (afferent) and motor (efferent) cytoplasmic processes of neurons in forming (A) a two-neuron and (B) a three-neuron reflex arc.

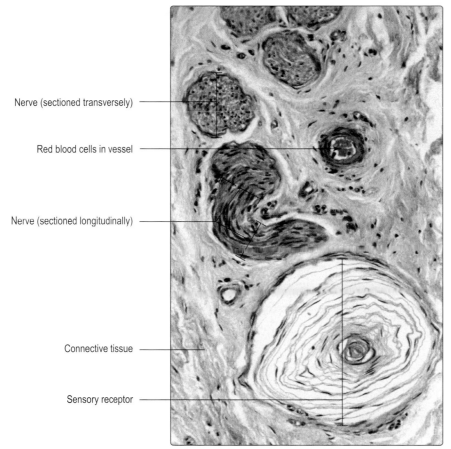

Fig. 6.11 **A sensory receptor (Pacinian corpuscle) and peripheral nerves (sectioned across their length and along their length).** Medium magnification.

choline and catecholamines such as noradrenaline and dopamine.

The arrival of a nerve (electrical) impulse at a synapse triggers the release of neurotransmitter molecules into the synaptic cleft. The neurotransmitters bind to the membrane of the postsynaptic cell and, if it is another nerve cell, a nerve (electrical) impulse is produced and transmitted by the postsynaptic neuron.

Synapses between axons and muscle cells are known as motor end plates (Fig. 6.13). Each axon usually branches at its peripheral end and forms synapses with several muscle cells. The presynaptic axonal membrane abuts the highly folded postsynaptic muscle cell membrane. The two membranes are separated by the synaptic cleft. The release of neurotransmitters triggers changes in the ionic permeability of the membrane of the muscle cells, which results in contraction. The motor neuron and the muscle cell (or cells) with which it synapses is described as a motor unit.

Ganglia and nuclei

Ganglia are defined as collections of neuronal perikarya (cell bodies) not in the CNS. The equivalent aggregations of neuronal perikarya in the CNS are known as nuclei. In addition to neuronal cell bodies, ganglia also contain supporting (satellite) cells and parts of the cytoplasmic processes (axons and dendrites) of neurons (Figs 6.3 and 6.14). The satellite cells surround and support the perikarya in ganglia by providing electrical insulation and ensuring that nutrients reach the neuronal perikarya. Connective tissue surrounds each ganglion and a sparse network of connective tissue is present within each (Fig. 6.3).

There are two types of ganglion:

- *Spinal ganglia* are attached to spinal nerves (Fig. 6.10) and located in intervertebral foramina. They are characterised by collections of closely packed sensory, pseudounipolar, neuronal perikarya. They receive and transmit signals about sensations through their single cytoplasmic process. Each cell body is surrounded by a layer of satellite cells (Fig. 6.14).
- *Autonomic ganglia* are part of the ANS and occupy sites near to the spinal cord (in pre- and paravertebral ganglia) and in the

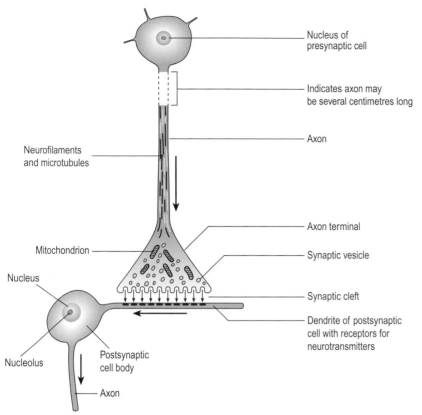

Nucleus of presynaptic cell

Indicates axon may be several centimetres long

Axon

Neurofilaments and microtubules

Axon terminal

Synaptic vesicle

Mitochondrion

Synaptic cleft

Nucleus

Dendrite of postsynaptic cell with receptors for neurotransmitters

Nucleolus

Postsynaptic cell body

Axon

Fig. 6.12 **The structure of an axo-dendritic synapse.** Arrows (large black) indicate the direction of travel of the nerve impulses.

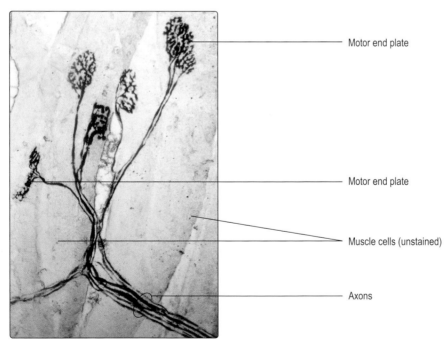

Motor end plate

Motor end plate

Muscle cells (unstained)

Axons

Fig. 6.13 **Motor end plates.** Special stain. Medium magnification.

walls of, or close to, some viscera. The neuronal cell bodies in autonomic ganglia are multipolar and receive signals, via synapses, from axons of preganglionic neurons. They transmit the signals away from ganglia via their axons.

Autonomic ganglia are classified into two functional types, sympathetic and parasympathetic.

- *Sympathetic ganglia.* The neurons in these ganglia are involved in the body's alarm responses (fright, fight and flight) and are in the sympathetic chain of paravertebral ganglia and in prevertebral ganglia.
- *Parasympathetic ganglia.* Parasympathetic neurons are involved in the 'rest and digest' activities of the body. They are similar in structure to sympathetic ganglia but are typically found in the walls of, or near to, the organs they affect (Fig. 6.15) and the number of perikarya present is often quite small.

Glial cells

Glial cells are present in the CNS and they are more numerous than the neurons. They function in maintenance, support and repair. There are three types: astrocytes, oligodendrocytes and microglial cells.

- *Astrocytes.* Each astrocyte has a small cell body with numerous, radiating, small cytoplasmic processes like stars, hence their name. They act in two ways. Firstly, they have cytoplasmic processes that are wrapped around blood vessels; this is an important structural and functional relationship forming the blood–brain barrier. This barrier prevents the passage of molecules larger than about 500 daltons between blood and brain. Secondly, they repair damaged tissue, a process known as gliosis. The latter is the equivalent of repair by fibroblasts in the rest of the body.
- *Oligodendrocytes.* These cells produce myelin which ensheaths some axons in the CNS.
- *Microglia.* These are small cells and they are the only nerve tissue cells which originate from mesoderm. In response to inflammation, they undergo phagocytosis and aid repair; in this they resemble macrophages (Chapters 4 and 8).

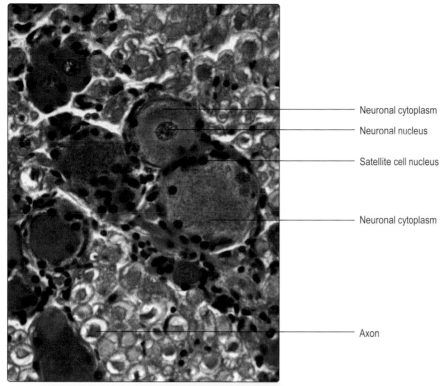

Fig. 6.14 **Ganglion.** Neuronal perikarya are surrounded by satellite cells. Many neuronal cytoplasmic processes are sectioned across their length. Lipid has been extracted from myelinated axons during processing and this appears as small spaces around some of the axons. Medium magnification.

Labels on figure 6.14:
- Neuronal cytoplasm
- Neuronal nucleus
- Satellite cell nucleus
- Neuronal cytoplasm
- Axon

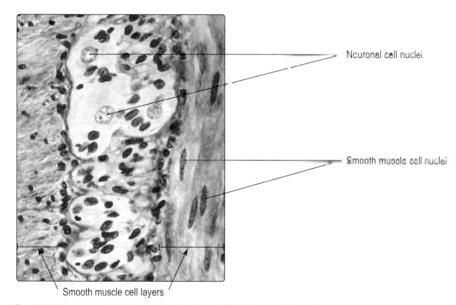

Fig. 6.15 **Parasympathetic ganglion in the wall of the small intestine.** These ganglion cells lie between two layers of smooth muscle. Connective tissue is stained blue. Special stain. Medium magnification.

Labels on figure 6.15:
- Neuronal cell nuclei
- Smooth muscle cell nuclei
- Smooth muscle cell layers

Brain and spinal cord

The arrangement of neurons in brain and spinal cord is complex (see Crossman AR, Neary D. *Neuroanatomy: An Illustrated Colour Text*, 3rd edn. Elsevier: 2005). Two principal areas are described in brain and spinal cord as white and grey matter. In the brain, grey matter forms the peripheral region, whereas in the spinal cord it is the central region (Fig. 6.10). Neuronal cell bodies are predominant in grey matter, and axons, particularly myelinated axons, are prominent in white matter. To the unaided eye, white matter appears white; it is the lipid content of myelin that gives this appearance. In histological sections the regions of grey and white matter can be clearly revealed (Fig. 6.16).

Peripheral nerves

Peripheral nerves pass between the CNS and the rest of the body. The peripheral nerves attached to the brain are known as cranial nerves and those attached to the spinal cord as spinal nerves. Peripheral nerves may be up to 2 cm in width and contain the cytoplasmic processes (axons and dendrites) of a very large number of neurons. Numerous ensheathing Schwann cells and connective tissue are also present. Peripheral nerves become smaller as they branch and pass around the body to the sites where the neuronal cell processes they contain initiate or receive signals. Their appearance in histological sections varies depending on the angle at which they are sectioned (Fig. 6.11). Individual cytoplasmic processes are difficult to distinguish in peripheral nerves but the nuclei of Schwann cells and supporting connective tissue cells can be seen, although not always distinguished (Fig. 6.11).

Peripheral nerves contain layers of connective tissue (Fig. 6.17). The connective tissue wraps around axons at three levels of organisation. Endoneurium surrounds individual axons. Groups of axons, with their coverings of endoneurium, are bundled together and surrounded by perineurium. The perineurium also packs the space between adjacent bundles of axons. Several bundles of axons within their investments of endoneurium and perineurium are surrounded by the connective tissue of the epineurium.

Most peripheral nerves contain neuronal cell processes which transmit impulses to the CNS and other cell processes which transmit impulses away from the CNS, respectively processes from afferent and efferent neurons. All peripheral nerves also carry cytoplasmic processes from sympathetic nerves, whereas some of those in the head and trunk also carry parasympathetic nerves.

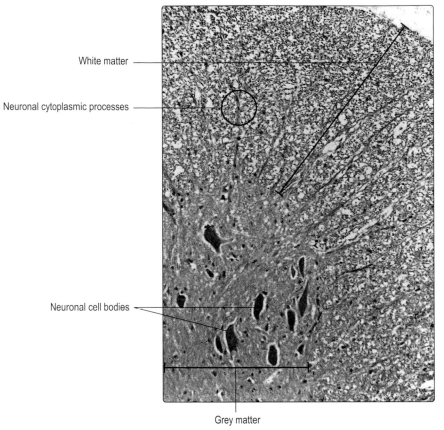

White matter

Neuronal cytoplasmic processes

Neuronal cell bodies

Grey matter

Fig. 6.16 **Grey and white matter of part of the spinal cord sectioned across its length.** Very low magnification.

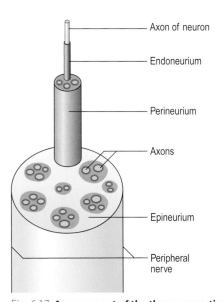

Axon of neuron

Endoneurium

Perineurium

Axons

Epineurium

Peripheral nerve

Fig. 6.17 **Arrangement of the three connective tissue layers around cytoplasmic processes of neurons (axons and dendrites) in a typical peripheral nerve.**

Summary

Nerve tissue
- consists of neurons (nerve cells), glial cells and satellite cells.

The nervous system comprises:
- the central nervous system (CNS) (brain and spinal cord)
- the peripheral nervous system (PNS) (nerve tissue not in the CNS).

The nervous system has two functional components:

- the somatic nervous system that detects sensations and controls the contraction of skeletal muscle
- the autonomic nervous system that controls the contraction of cardiac and smooth muscle and the secretory activity of many glands.

Neurons
- Neurons mostly have large cell bodies (perikarya) with granular cytoplasm owing to RER involved in protein synthesis.
- They have cytoplasmic processes (usually many dendrites which transmit nerve (electrical) impulses to their perikaryon and a single axon which transmits signals away from the perikaryon).
- They transmit impulses fastest along axons ensheathed in myelin formed by Schwann cells in the PNS and oligodendrocytes in the CNS.
- Sensory signals are transmitted by afferent neurons to the CNS and efferent neurons carry impulses away from the CNS which affect the function of, for example, muscles.

Synapses
- These are specialised junctions between neurons or between neurons and other cell types.
  - A nerve impulse reaching a synapse stimulates the release of neurotransmitter molecules into the synaptic cleft between the pre- and postsynaptic cells. Neurotransmitters stimulate the postsynaptic cells to transmit a nerve impulse (if they are neurons), or to contract (if they are muscle cells), or to secrete or to stop secreting (if they are gland cells).

Ganglia and nuclei
- Ganglia are groups of neuronal cells bodies in the PNS; nuclei are collections of neuronal cell bodies in the CNS.
- Spinal ganglia are part of the somatic nervous system.
- Autonomic ganglia are part of the autonomic nervous system. Sympathetic ganglia are involved in fright, fight and flight responses. Parasympathetic ganglia are involved in rest and digest activities.

Types of glial cell
- Astrocytes are small cells involved in forming a structural and functional barrier between the blood and the brain.
- Oligodendrocytes form myelin sheaths around some axons in the CNS.
- Microglia are able to aid repair of damaged tissue.

Chapter 7
The skin

Skin is considered to be the largest organ. It covers the whole surface of the body and is continuous at entry and exits points of the body with the mucous membranes lining the nose, mouth and anus, and the reproductive and urinary openings. Skin on the eyelids is replaced on the inner surfaces of the lids by the moist epithelium of the conjunctiva. At the ear the skin continues into the external acoustic meatus and is continuous with the tympanic membrane which separates the outer ear from the middle ear.

All four types of primary tissue (epithelial, connective, muscle and nerve) are present in the skin and its functions are related to its structure. The skin has roles in protection against microbes, physical and chemical damage and UV radiation; it also prevents excess water loss. Skin plays an important role in regulating body temperature by the ability of sweat glands to secrete sweat onto the surface of the skin which cools the body as it evaporates. In addition, the amount of blood flowing in vessels in the skin varies and this too helps in regulating heat loss and thus body temperature. Skin also has important roles as a sense organ detecting stimuli through specific sensory nerve receptors. In addition, cells in the surface of skin exposed to sunlight are involved in the production of vitamin D.

The skin consists of two layers: the superficial epidermis (the epithelium of skin) and the deeper dermis consisting mainly of connective tissue (Figs 7.1 and 7.2). The dermis is superficial to the hypodermis and the latter is not considered to be part of the skin. The hypodermis is composed mainly of connective tissue, which may contain large numbers of adipose cells; the hypodermis is also known as superficial fascia or subcutaneous tissue.

Epidermis

The epidermis is derived from the ectoderm germ layer of the embryo and is composed of a stratified, squamous, keratinised epithelium (Figs 7.2 and 7.3). It is made up of keratinocytes, the protein keratin and other specialised cell types (see below). Extending through the epidermis in many regions of the body are hairs (see below) and spiral channels which end as pores and allow for the passage of sweat (Fig. 7.3).

The epidermis may be described in five layers, though all layers are present only in thick skin, such as on the palms of the hand and soles of the feet.

- *Stratum corneum.* This is the most superficial layer and consists of the protein keratin; no cells are present. In thick skin (Fig. 7.3) the keratin is in numerous layers; there is less keratin in thin skin (Fig. 7.2). Keratin is a filamentous protein produced by keratinocytes in deeper layers of the epidermis. It confers toughness and protection on the epidermis and helps to prevent water loss and dehydration of cells in the epidermis (and deeper). Some keratinocytes in deeper layers produce lipids which are added to the stratum corneum,

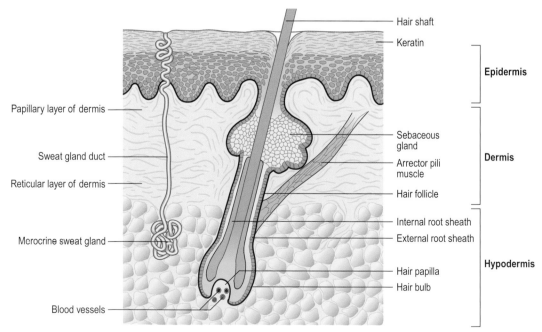

Fig. 7.1 **The structure of skin, including a hair follicle, sebaceous and sweat glands and an arrector pili muscle.**

Fig. 7.2 **Skin (thin).** At the junction of the epidermis and the connective tissue (green) of the dermis interdigitations occur which help bind the layers together. The interdigitations may be ridges or papillae; only by examining adjacent sections would their three-dimensional shape be revealed. Small blood vessels in the dermis supply oxygen and nutrients to the epidermis. Special stain. Medium magnification.

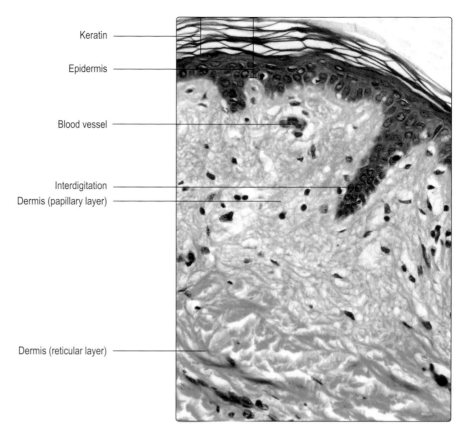

Keratin

Epidermis

Blood vessel

Interdigitation
Dermis (papillary layer)

Dermis (reticular layer)

Fig. 7.3 **Skin (thick).** A sweat gland duct passes sweat from a sweat gland (not shown) to a pore on the surface of the skin via a spiralling channel in the keratin. Low magnification.

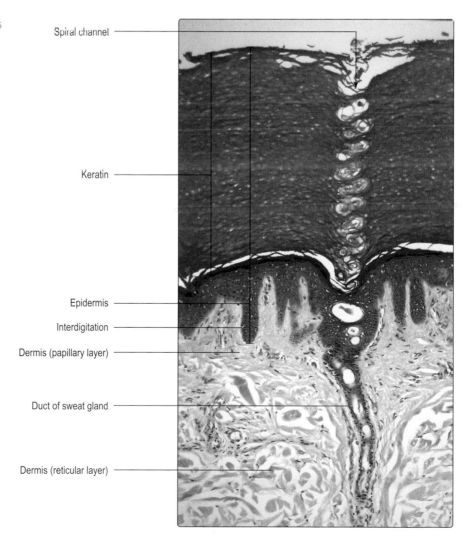

Spiral channel

Keratin

Epidermis
Interdigitation
Dermis (papillary layer)

Duct of sweat gland

Dermis (reticular layer)

and this increases the ability of skin to resist water absorption. The surface of the stratum corneum is constantly being shed, particularly if it is subjected to abrasion. Importantly, the stratum corneum is constantly being added to as cells in the deeper layers move towards the surface at a rate which equals the rate at which the keratin is shed.

■ *Stratum lucidum*. This is a thin layer of keratinocytes, adjacent to the stratum corneum, that are at the end stage of their lives. The cells are packed with keratin and do not possess nuclei or organelles. They lose their cell membrane and become the basal layer of the stratum corneum. The change is rapid and the layer is seen only in the thickest skin.

■ *Stratum granulosum*. This layer may be up to five cells deep, but in thin skin it may be absent. It is characterised by the presence of cytoplasmic granules of keratohyalin (Fig. 7.4). Other cytoplasmic granules contain lipids and these are released into extracellular spaces and confer waterproofing on the superficial layers of the epidermis. Upper cells in this stratum die and then become part of the stratum lucidum.

■ *Stratum spinosum*. This is the thickest layer of the epidermis, and is characterised by the presence of 'prickle' cells (Fig. 7.4). The angular appearance of these keratinocytes in sectioned material is due to the large number of desmosomes between adjacent keratinocytes, which are important in holding the cells together and resisting shearing forces. Increasing amounts of cytoplasmic keratin filaments are produced by keratinocytes in this layer. The uppermost cells in this layer develop keratohyalin granules, move towards the surface and become part of the stratum granulosum.

■ *Stratum germinativum*. This is the deepest layer of the epidermis and consists of cuboidal epithelial cells (Fig. 7.4). The basal cells in the stratum germinativum are attached to the basement membrane of the epidermis, which, in turn, is adjacent to the dermis. The cells in this stratum undergo mitosis and are the stem cells of the epidermis. Some offspring cells remain in this layer, undergo further mitotic activity, and thus continue as stem cells. Other offspring cells begin to produce keratin filaments and migrate towards the surface of the epidermis; this initially replaces the keratinocytes in the stratum spinosum. Over a period of about 30 days, keratinocytes produced by mitosis in the stratum germinativum migrate towards the surface of skin, die and the keratin they have formed is shed.

Within the epidermis there are various cell types in addition to keratinocytes.

■ *Merkel cells*. These cells are scattered throughout the stratum germinativum and are thought to act as mechanoreceptors.

■ *Langerhans cells*. These cells are derived from bone marrow cells and they have an immunological function (Chapter 8). They are mainly located in the stratum spinosum.

■ *Melanocytes*. These cells produce pigment and are present in the stratum germinativum between the mitotically active cells. Melanin is responsible for giving skin a brownish colour and carotene for giving it a yellowish colour. The type and amount of pigment present is affected by the genetic make-up of the individual and, in the case of melanin, the amount of exposure to ultraviolet light (sunlight stimulates the synthesis and spread of melanin). Melanocytes have long cytoplasmic processes in which the melanin granules are present. They

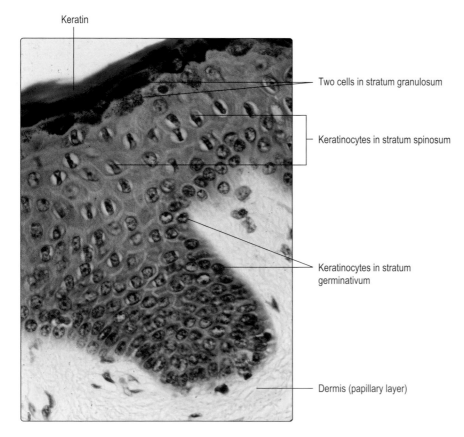

Keratin

Two cells in stratum granulosum

Keratinocytes in stratum spinosum

Keratinocytes in stratum germinativum

Dermis (papillary layer)

Fig. 7.4 **Skin.** As keratohyalin granules accumulate in cells in the stratum granulosum they obscure structural detail; early stages with few distinct granules and later stages are present. Keratinocytes in the stratum spinosum appear to be surrounded by thin, palely stained regions and have a 'prickly' appearance with angular outlines. High magnification.

also pass melanin to keratinocytes. The melanin is often located in the cytoplasm of keratinocytes between the nucleus and the surface of the skin (Fig. 7.5); there, it helps protect DNA from damage by UV light.

Dermis

The dermis is derived from the mesoderm layer of the embryo and consists largely of connective tissue fibres and cells. Also present in the dermis are structures which may extend between the hypodermis and the epidermis, e.g. parts of developing hairs in hair follicles, sebaceous glands and sweat glands (see below). The dermis is divided into two layers, the papillary and the reticular layer.

- *Papillary layer.* This is the most superficial layer and it interdigitates with the epidermis through a series of dermal ridges and papillae (Figs 7.2 and 7.3). In this way, the

attachment of the epidermis and the dermis is strengthened. The papillary layer is characterised by loose connective tissue, including collagen, reticulin and elastin fibres and fibroblasts. There are also the transient cell types typical of connective tissue, e.g. white blood cells (Chapters 4 and 8). In the papillary region there are blood vessels that supply oxygen and nutrients to nearby cells, including epidermal cells, and that are also involved in temperature regulation. Some sensory nerve endings are present in the papillary region of the dermis.

- *Reticular layer.* The reticular layer is deep to the papillary layer but the border between them is a gradual transition: it connects the skin to the underlying hypodermis. Dense, irregular connective tissue (Figs 7.2 and 7.3) containing many collagen fibres is predominant in the reticular layer. The transient cell population is less abundant in the reticular layer

than in the papillary layer.

Glands of skin

Exocrine glands are present in skin. Some secrete sweat and are involved in temperature regulation. Others, sebaceous glands, secrete lipids and most are associated with hairs. In females, modified glands in the skin (mammary glands) are able to secrete milk in response to the hormones present during and after pregnancy (Chapter 16).

Sweat glands

- *Merocrine sweat glands.* These are present in skin (Figs 7.1 and 7.6) all over the body and they are simple, coiled tubular glands (Chapter 3). The secretory cells are located deep in the dermis, and even in the underlying hypodermis. An epithelial lined duct (Fig. 7.3) drains each gland and it passes to the superficial layer of the epidermis (stratum corneum). The duct is replaced by a spiral channel through the stratum corneum (Fig. 7.3) and opens at a pore on the surface of the skin. Merocrine sweat glands are innervated by sympathetic nerves and may be stimulated to secrete under conditions of stress, as well as in order to cool the body. Myoepithelial cells surrounding the gland cells contract and assist in the expulsion of sweat.
- *Apocrine sweat glands.* This type of sweat gland is present in the axilla, around nipples and in the anal region. The glands are larger than merocrine sweat glands, and they are located more deeply in the dermis and underlying hypodermis. Unlike merocrine glands, apocrine sweat glands do not secrete onto the surface of the skin; instead, they secrete around developing hairs in hair follicles. Secretion by apocrine sweat glands is influenced by sex hormones, and, after bacterial action, their secretions have a characteristic odour. It is thought that this odour may impart pheromone-like qualities to the secretion.

Sebaceous glands

- *Sebaceous glands* (Figs 7.1 and 7.7) secrete a lipid-based substance known as sebum. They release their secretions by the holocrine method and as the cells die the sebum is

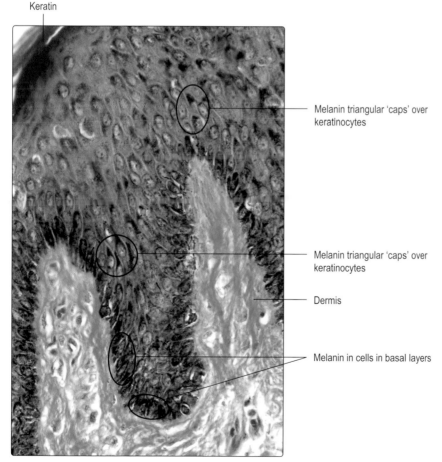

Keratin

Melanin triangular 'caps' over keratinocytes

Melanin triangular 'caps' over keratinocytes

Dermis

Melanin in cells in basal layers

Fig. 7.5 **Skin (pigmented with melanin).** Melanin is visible in some of the keratinocytes 'capping' the nucleus and forming a barrier to UV light. The melanin is formed in melanocytes in basal layers although the precise identity of these cells is not revealed at this magnification. Special stain. High magnification.

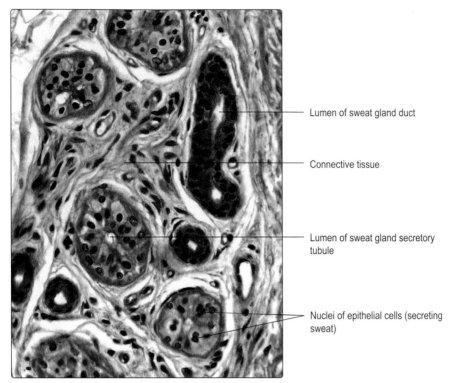

Fig. 7.6 **Sweat gland.** Secretory epithelial cells lining the coiled tube forming a sweat gland appear palely stained with eosin in comparison with the cells lining the ducts. Connective tissue supports the epithelial cells forming the gland. High magnification.

- Lumen of sweat gland duct
- Connective tissue
- Lumen of sweat gland secretory tubule
- Nuclei of epithelial cells (secreting sweat)

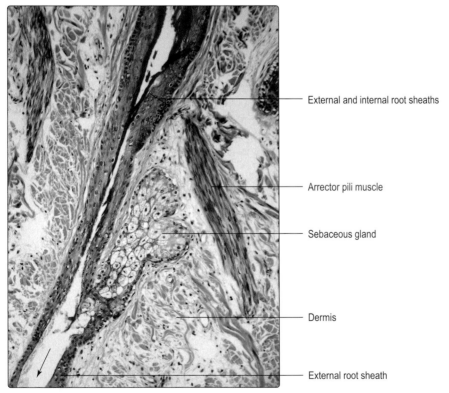

Fig. 7.7 **Part of a hair follicle, sebaceous gland and smooth muscle cells.** The developing hair has been lost during processing. The space it occupied and an arrow shows the direction along which it would have grown. Connective tissue is stained green. Special stain. Medium magnification.

- External and internal root sheaths
- Arrector pili muscle
- Sebaceous gland
- Dermis
- External root sheath

released from the cytoplasm and empty spaces may be apparent in the gland. The activity of sebaceous glands is influenced by sex hormones and their secretory activity increases substantially after puberty. In areas where there are hairs, sebaceous glands secrete into the follicle of each hair (see below) and the sebum 'conditions' the hair. In locations where there are no hairs (e.g. the palms and soles) sebaceous glands open directly onto the surface of the skin and help maintain its texture and condition.

Hair follicles

Hair is formed largely of a compact, dense form of keratin. Each hair is produced in a structure known as a hair follicle (Fig. 7.1). Hairs are widespread over the body surface though they are absent from the palms, soles, parts of the genitalia, tips of fingers and toes, and lips. Hairs are of two types: vellus hairs, which are the short, fine, soft hairs on the skin, and terminal hairs, which are the long hairs such as on the scalp. Hairs may be coloured, e.g. by the presence of a pigment such as melanin.

Hair follicles develop as cylindrical invaginations of the epidermis and they extend into the dermis and, in some instances, also into the hypodermis. Straight hair grows from straight follicles, and spiralling follicles give rise to curly hairs. Hair follicles are surrounded by connective tissue (Fig. 7.8). During the growing phase of a hair the base of its follicle is expanded into a bulbous portion (Figs 7.8 and 7.9). Cell proliferation in the epidermal-like cells of the bulb produces a variety of cells. Some of these cells form part of the follicle and move towards the surface and others, centrally placed, form the hair which grows out from the follicle. Pigment such as melanin in cells in this region (Fig. 7.9) affect the colour of the hair. Each hair bulb is invaginated by a dermal papilla of connective tissue (Fig. 7.9) containing blood vessels which are essential for hair growth.

Each hair follicle is lined by layers of cells similar to epidermal cells, and by cells produced by mitosis of cells in the hair bulb. The outer layers of epidermal-like cells are known as the external root sheath (Figs 7.1 and 7.9). An inner sheath, formed by cells produced in the hair bulb, extends only part way along the follicle. It is the innermost cells within the inner sheath which undergo keratinisation and form the hair shaft. At the region where the inner sheath stops, secretions from sebaceous glands drain into the follicle (Fig. 7.7) and coat the hair as it grows out of the follicle.

Hair growth is cyclical. Growth in length usually occurs for several years and then the follicle enters a rest phase when mitosis in the bulb region stops and the bulb shrinks in size. In the rest phase, the hair eventually falls

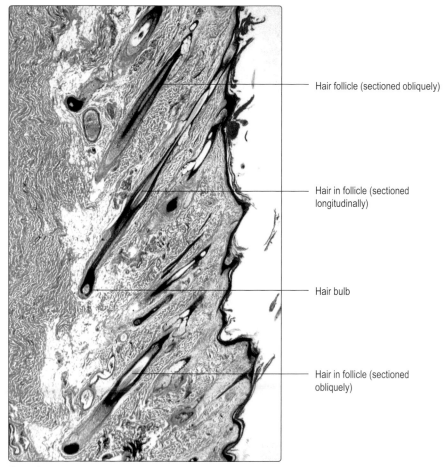

Fig. 7.8 **Hair.** Several hair follicles have been sectioned, only one along its length from the hair bulb to the surface. Hair appears yellowish and keratin of the stratum corneum reddish. Connective tissue is stained green. Special stain. Very low magnification.

Labels for Fig. 7.8:
- Hair follicle (sectioned obliquely)
- Hair in follicle (sectioned longitudinally)
- Hair bulb
- Hair in follicle (sectioned obliquely)

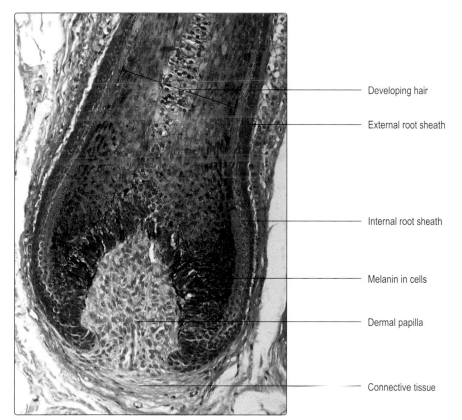

Fig. 7.9 **Hair bulb.** Melanocytes are present among the epithelial cells in the bulb and melanin can be distinguished as dark brown material. (The precise detail of melanin in cells is not seen at this magnification.) Connective tissue of the dermis extends as a papilla into the hair bulb. Special stain. Medium magnification.

Labels for Fig. 7.9:
- Developing hair
- External root sheath
- Internal root sheath
- Melanin in cells
- Dermal papilla
- Connective tissue

out of the follicle and, after several weeks, mitosis in the bulb begins and this new growth phase produces another hair.

Muscles, nerves and blood vessels in the dermis and hypodermis

Smooth muscle cells, known as arrectores pilorum, are associated with hair follicles and their sebaceous glands (Figs 7.1 and 7.7). The muscle cells lie obliquely and attach the hair follicle to connective tissue in the dermis. Sympathetic nerves stimulate contraction of these smooth muscle cells and this causes hairs to 'stand on end'. Sympathetic nerves also supply sweat glands and the smooth muscle cells in the walls of blood vessels in the skin. The flow of blood through vessels in skin and the amount of sweat secreted varies, particularly as a means of maintaining body temperature by varying heat loss from the body. Other nerves in skin transmit sensory information to the CNS. There are several types of nerve ending in skin that may be distinguished by their morphology and these include free nerve endings, Pacinian corpuscles, Meissner's corpuscles and Merkel cells. The free nerve endings detect pain and temperature changes. Pacinian corpuscles (Chapter 6, Fig. 6.11) have a characteristic lamellated appearance enclosing a central nerve ending and they detect pressure changes. Meissner's corpuscles are located in dermal papillae and detect touch. Merkel cells also detect touch and are located in the epidermis.

Clinical notes

Psoriasis This is a condition in which there is overproliferation of keratinocytes. This results in patches of thick, silvery, scaly lesions particularly on the scalp, knees and elbows. The cause is unknown.

Age With age, numerous changes occur in skin. In particular, elastin fibres disappear so the skin loses the ability to recoil after being stretched. The epidermis becomes thinner with age and less able to withstand trauma.

Tumours Tumours of the skin may be benign or malignant. Of the benign tumours, warts (papillomata) are common. Warts occur at any site, and are simple proliferations of epidermal cells resulting from infection of the keratinocytes with a papilloma virus. Basal cell carcinomas of skin are common neoplasms which rarely spread to distant sites. However, they spread into the dermis and can cause damage in the local region. Of all the skin tumours the most malignant are malignant melanomas (neoplasms of melanocytes) and they often have fatal consequences.

Summary

Skin:

- is an organ covering the body and consists of epidermis and dermis
- is involved in protection against physical trauma, dehydration, ultraviolet light, harmful molecules and microorganisms
- aids control of body temperature
    - by secretion of sweat and variation in blood flow through blood vessels near the surface of the skin
- has sensory nerve receptors
- is involved in producing vitamin D.

The epidermis is a stratified, squamous, keratinised epithelium:

- the basal layer of cells (keratinocytes) act as stem cells
- keratinocytes move from the basal layer, differentiate, make keratin and die, and keratin is shed
- other cells in the epithelium make pigment, others are involved in immune responses.

The dermis consists mainly of connective tissue cells and fibres:

- it has a papillary layer adjacent to the epidermis and a denser, reticular layer adjacent to the hypodermis.

Sweat glands (in most regions of the body):

- consist of secretory cells lining coiled tubes in the dermis or hypodermis
- secrete sweat by the merocrine method under the influence of sympathetic nerves and aid the regulation of body temperature.

Sebaceous glands synthesise and secrete lipids forming sebum:

- secretion occurs by the holocrine method and is affected by sex hormones
- most secretions coat developing hairs.

Hair:

- is a compact, dense form of keratin and develops in a hair follicle
    - follicles extend between the surface of skin and the dermis or hypodermis
    - actively growing hair follicles have mitotically active cells at the base
    - cells move from the base towards the skin surface, some form the hair
    - smooth muscle attached to hair follicles, under control of sympathetic nerves, can make hairs 'stand on end'.

Chapter 8
The blood and immune system

Blood and the immune system contain a wide variety of cells and carry out diverse functions. All the components of blood and the immune system may be considered as connective tissue and the vast majority of the cells is derived from mesoderm. Blood flows around the body in tubes known as blood vessels (Chapter 10) and is involved in moving cells and molecules. Tissue fluid (extracellular fluid), which bathes many of the cells in the body, is the aqueous component of extracellular matrix (Chapter 4) and is formed from blood. The immune system protects the body from invasion and damage by microorganisms and from many potentially harmful molecules. This system recognises cells and molecules 'foreign' to the body and generates immune cells and molecules in defensive immune responses. The immune system involves a wide variety of cells and molecules including non-specialised and specialised cells and molecules which carry out immune responses. The molecules vary in size and type but many are large protein molecules such as antibodies which react specifically with other molecules (antigens). Blood plays a major role in transporting immune cells and antibodies around the body.

The cellular components of the immune system, as well as circulating in blood, are widely distributed throughout organs of the body and are predominant in specialised organs (e.g. the thymus and spleen). Immune cells are also present in large numbers in lymph nodes, structures which are integral parts of the circulatory system that return excess tissue fluid to blood (see below and Chapter 10). Localised clusters of immune cells are present in other regions of the body, particularly where mucosal surfaces are exposed to harmful molecules and organisms in the environment (e.g. substances ingested into the digestive tract or breathed into the respiratory tract).

Blood

Blood consists of cells and parts of cells suspended in a fluid, the plasma. The cellular components of blood are red and white blood cells (respectively, erythrocytes and leucocytes) and parts of cells, platelets (thrombocytes). Plasma is a straw-coloured fluid that contains electrolytes, carbohydrates, lipids and proteins (including albumin and globulins); however, plasma is mainly water. Erythrocytes constitute just over 40% of blood volume with just 1% leucocytes; most of the rest is plasma.

Although blood is considered to be a form of connective tissue in which the extracellular matrix is the fluid plasma, the function of blood differs from the functions of other forms of connective tissue. Blood circulates via the cardiovascular system and delivers oxygen and various molecules, including nutrients and hormones, to cells of the body. Blood also facilitates the removal of waste molecules from body tissues, including carbon dioxide. Importantly, blood is able to coagulate and prevent excessive blood loss if blood vessels are damaged.

The ability of blood to deliver molecules to and remove other molecules from the body is facilitated by blood forming tissue fluid (extracellular fluid). Some of the plasma fluid (and the smaller molecules it contains) leaves blood vessels via the endothelial cells lining small blood vessels and bathes surrounding cells in tissue fluid. White blood cells also leave small blood vessels and these are particularly important in the defence mechanisms provided by the immune system. Some tissue fluid and white blood cells eventually return to blood via a series of lymphatic vessels and lymph nodes (see below).

Blood cells

Blood cells in routine histological sections may be identified as individual cells. However, in many instances details of individual blood cells may not readily be distinguished (Fig. 8.1). To study blood cells in detail it is usual to spread blood onto a glass microscope slide, a process which makes a 'blood smear'. Smears display the whole of the cells as opposed to cells in histological sections which may have been sliced during preparation (and show only part of individual cells).

Erythrocytes (red blood cells)

An erythrocyte is a membrane-bound cytoplasmic structure which does not have a nucleus. Erythrocytes lose their nuclei during their formation in bone marrow, just before they are released into blood vessels. Mature erythrocytes are biconcave discs approximately 7 μm in diameter but are easily distorted and are able to pass along narrow blood vessels about 3.5 μm in diameter. Identifying red blood cells and knowing their maximum diameter can be used as a scale for assessing the size of other features in histological specimens (Fig. 8.1). In blood smears, erythrocytes usually appear rounded and many have palely stained centres reflecting their central, thinner region of cytoplasm (Figs 8.2–8.4).

Erythrocytes transport oxygen from the lungs to the other parts of the body. The majority of their cytoplasm is made up of the iron-containing protein haemoglobin and only a few organelles (mitochondria and ribosomes) are present. Erythrocytes are referred to as red blood cells because the iron of haemoglobin confers the red colour on blood. Oxygen has a high affinity for the iron in haemoglobin in locations where there is a high oxygen concentration, such as the lungs. In regions with relatively low oxygen concentrations, such as in most body regions other than the lungs, the oxygen is liberated and used in metabolic processes. The reverse is true of carbon dioxide, a waste product of glucose metabolism. It is the globin (the protein component of haemo-

Fig. 8.1 **Liver.** The red blood cells in some blood vessels can be identified as individual structures and the largest diameter taken as 7 μm. In other vessels, individual red blood cells cannot be distinguished but they stain a similar shade of red with eosin. White blood cells in blood vessels in sections at this magnification can be identified only by their densely stained nuclei. Plasma proteins fixed in the lumen of the large vessel stain lightly with eosin. Medium magnification.

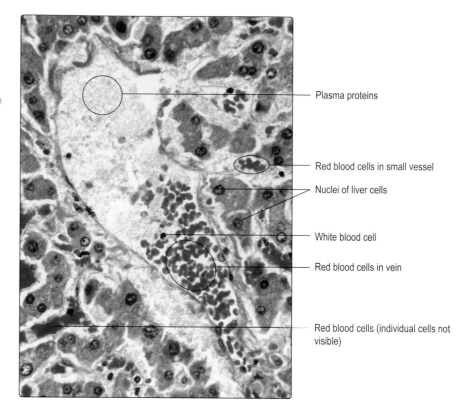

Plasma proteins

Red blood cells in small vessel

Nuclei of liver cells

White blood cell

Red blood cells in vein

Red blood cells (individual cells not visible)

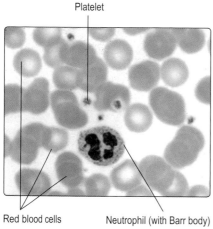

Platelet

Red blood cells   Neutrophil (with Barr body)

Fig. 8.2 **Blood smear.** Red blood cells, neutrophil, platelets. Special stain. Very high magnification.

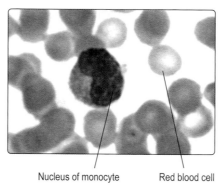

Nucleus of monocyte   Red blood cell

Fig. 8.4 **Blood smear.** Red blood cells, monocyte. Special stain. Very high magnification.

globin) that carries some of the carbon dioxide from body tissues to the lungs.

Erythrocytes have a life span of approximately 120 days and after this time they are destroyed by cells in the liver, spleen and bone marrow, probably because they become less able to change shape. The rate of production of new erythrocytes from the bone marrow normally equals the rate at which they are destroyed. Any loss of blood from the circulation, as a result of trauma for example, is followed by an increase in the production of erythrocytes and their release into circulation until normal numbers in blood are restored.

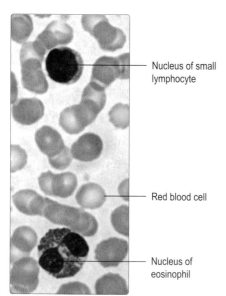

Nucleus of small lymphocyte

Red blood cell

Nucleus of eosinophil

Fig. 8.3 **Blood smear.** Red blood cells, eosinophil, small lymphocyte. Special stain. Very high magnification.

Clinical note

Anaemia This common blood disorder occurs when there is not enough haemoglobin to supply oxygen to support the metabolic requirements of the body's cells. An anaemic person may look pale, feel weak and easily become short of breath. The most common cause of anaemia is a shortage of iron, the element essential for the formation and function of haemoglobin. Excessively heavy blood loss, e.g. at menstruation, may be a cause of anaemia as enough iron may not be available to support red blood cell production at a rate which replaces the losses, particularly if the losses have occurred repeatedly over many months.

Other types of anaemia have a genetic basis. For example, in sickle cell anaemia the haemoglobin molecule is abnormal. In regions of the body in which oxygen levels are low the haemoglobin molecule becomes rigid and the red blood cells become less flexible and take on the shape of a sickle. As a result, many red blood cells die prematurely in the spleen or they may block small vessels around the body. Life expectancy is likely to be considerably reduced.

Leucocytes (white blood cells)

Leucocytes are referred to as white blood cells because of their whitish or buff colour in the zone between plasma and red blood cells after centrifugation of blood (a process used to determine the proportion of red cells in blood). Leucocytes are categorised by their content of cytoplasmic granules and by their nuclear morphology. Leucocytes with granules are known as granulocytes and their nuclei have two or more lobes. Granulocytes are subdivided into three categories by the affinity of their granules for certain dyes. Leucocytes without granules are known as agranulocytes. There are two categories of agranulocyte: lymphocytes, which each have a spherical nucleus, and monocytes, which each have an indented, spherical nucleus.

Granulocytes

- *Neutrophils.* These constitute about 70% of the total leucocyte population in peripheral blood. Neutrophils are also known as polymorphonuclear leucocytes (PMNLs) because each has a multilobed nucleus (Fig. 8.2). The nuclei of neutrophils in females are characterised by the possession of a Barr body (Fig. 8.2), which is manifest as a small drumstick projection from one of the lobes of the nucleus. Barr bodies represent the inactive second X chromosome of females, but they are seen on only a small proportion of neutrophil nuclei. The granules of neutrophils do not stain with acidic or basic dyes. Some of the granules are very small and not readily seen by light microscopy. Some are lysosomes and the enzymes they contain are typical of lysosomes, e.g. acid phosphatase.

  Neutrophils develop in bone marrow, enter blood vessels and thus circulate around the body. However, they migrate out of blood vessels within a few days and move rapidly through body tissues where normally they die after a few days. If neutrophils encounter bacteria they are able to engulf and kill them. They kill bacteria by a variety of mechanisms, one of which involves hydrogen peroxide. Neutrophils that have performed their killing function die and accumulate in pus at the site of the infection. If the infection persists, large numbers of neutrophils leave blood and are attracted to the site(s) of infection and large numbers are also released into circulation from the bone marrow.

- *Eosinophils.* An eosinophil is characterised by its bi-lobed nucleus and by numerous granules which stain heavily pink with eosin and with the staining methods for examining blood smears (Fig. 8.3). Lysosomes are also present in eosinophils. Eosinophils develop in bone marrow and normally constitute 2–4% of the leucocytes present in peripheral blood. Eosinophils function by their ability to respond to antigen–antibody complexes and to parasites. Their granules release their contents which bind to, and kill, parasites. They are able to phagocytose and digest antigen–antibody complexes and the remains of parasites. In addition, they release antihistamines that reduce the inflammatory processes that are initiated by such complexes and organisms. Eosinophils are present in increased numbers in blood and body tissues during allergic reactions, such as hay fever, and in response to infections by parasites.

- *Basophils.* The granules of basophils are stained by basic dyes such as haematoxylin. The nuclei of basophils are bi-lobed but the granules are often so numerous that they obscure the rest of the cytoplasm and the nucleus in blood smears. Basophils develop in bone marrow and they constitute only 0.5–1% of the total leucocyte population in peripheral blood. They leave the blood and are involved in initiating inflammatory reactions.

Agranulocytes

- *Lymphocytes.* These make up 20–30% of the total number of leucocytes circulating in blood. Lymphocytes are also present in bone marrow, thymus, spleen and lymph nodes, and in lymphoid regions in other organs, e.g. in parts of the gastrointestinal, urinary, reproductive and respiratory tracts. Some lymphocytes develop in bone marrow but others are produced in the thymus and at other sites in the body in response to immune stimuli. In general, lymphocytes function at such sites, and not in peripheral blood.

  Lymphocytes may be described as small, medium or large. Small lymphocytes make up about 95% of the lymphocytes in peripheral blood and they are distinguished by having a densely stained nucleus that occupies the bulk of the cell (Fig. 8.3). Lymphocytes responding to an immune stimulus are larger than small lymphocytes and have relatively more cytoplasm – they are described as medium or large lymphocytes.

  Lymphocytes are also categorised according to their function. Their morphology does not distinguish the functional types but categories can be identified by using labelled antibodies to identify specific molecules on their cell membrane. The categories are B lymphocytes, T lymphocytes and natural killer (NK) cells.

- *B lymphocytes* constitute 5–15% of small lymphocytes in peripheral blood. They migrate out of blood vessels and through body tissues and respond to antigenic stimulation by increasing in size and differentiating into plasma cells (see below).
- *T lymphocytes* constitute 65–75% of small lymphocytes in peripheral blood. They are small when they are inactive but differentiate into larger lymphocytes when responding to immune stimulation. T lymphocytes are responsible for cell-mediated immunity, which is the type of cellular immune response engaged in detecting foreign cells and destroying them. This involves T lymphocytes detecting certain molecules which may be on the surface of foreign cells, or on the body's own cells that have become abnormal (e.g. malignant or infected by virus). This recognition stimulates the T lymphocytes to divide and increases the number of T lymphocytes able to attack specifically and destroy 'foreign' cells. T lymphocytes also produce a variety of molecular signals that regulate other cells involved in mounting immune responses.
- *Natural killer (NK) cells* comprise 10–15% of the lymphocytes in peripheral blood. They are larger cells than small lymphocytes and they have a few granules in their cytoplasm. NK cells migrate through body tissues and have the ability to detect and kill foreign cells. Their activity is regulated by factors produced by subsets of T lymphocytes.

- Monocytes. Monocytes are derived from precursor cells in bone marrow and constitute about 5% of the leucocytes in blood. They are 15–20 µm in diameter and their nucleus appears indented in smears (Fig. 8.4). Monocytes leave blood vessels, migrate through tissues and become macrophages (see below).

Platelets (thrombocytes)

Platelets (Fig. 8.2) are cytoplasmic fragments of megakaryocytes, a large cell type present in bone marrow (see below). Platelets are released into blood vessels in bone marrow and they then circulate around the body. Platelets are essential for blood clotting and help control haemorrhage.

Other cells involved in immune responses

Mast cells

Mast cells are present in connective tissues of the body and they are densely packed with granules which may hide the nucleus (Fig. 8.5). They resemble the basophils in blood. Mast cells have receptors for a type of antibody (immunoglobulin E) on their cell membranes and these antibodies are produced in response to allergen(s). A subsequent exposure to the same allergen(s) causes the mast cells to release histamine (a vasoactive molecule which affects the diameter of blood vessels) from their granules as well as other mediators of the inflammatory response. This type of reaction can be rapid and fatal and is known as an anaphylactic reaction.

Plasma cells

Plasma cells are often evident at sites of infection associated with chronic inflammation and in lymph nodes (see below). They are the end stage of differentiation of B lymphocytes and they mount a humoral immune response by producing specific antibodies (e.g. immunoglobulins A and G) to specific antigens. Plasma cells may appear ovoid in shape, are larger than the B lymphocytes and are identified by the eccentric position of their nucleus (Fig. 8.6). The cytoplasm of each plasma cell has large amounts of rough endoplasmic reticulum synthesising a particular immunoglobulin which functions as a specific antibody. The antibody molecules are released from plasma cells and circulate in tissue fluids, lymph and peripheral blood where they are able to react with their specific antigen(s).

> ### Clinical note
>
> **White blood cell disorders** Increased numbers of normal neutrophils in peripheral blood or other areas of the body may be due to a bacterial infection whereas increased numbers of eosinophils may be due to a parasitic infection or to an allergic reaction.
>
> Leukaemias result from the proliferation of malignant white blood cells in the bone marrow. Large numbers of white blood cells, which may appear normal or abnormal, enter peripheral blood. Leukaemias are classified according to the type of white cell produced in high numbers (granulocyte, lymphocyte or monocyte) and whether the progress of the disease can be described as chronic or acute. Chronic leukaemias progress slowly, but in acute leukaemias the disease process progresses rapidly and many of the cells released into the bloodstream appear immature or grossly abnormal.

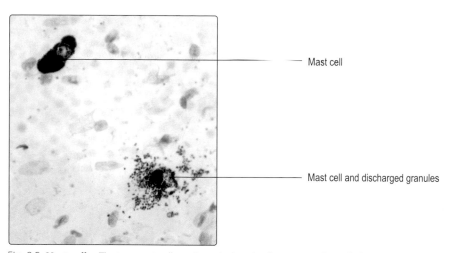

Fig. 8.5 **Mast cells.** The two mast cells are intensively stained amongst other cells (connective and epithelial) which are revealed only by their palely stained nuclei. One mast cell has discharged its granules. Special stain. High magnification.

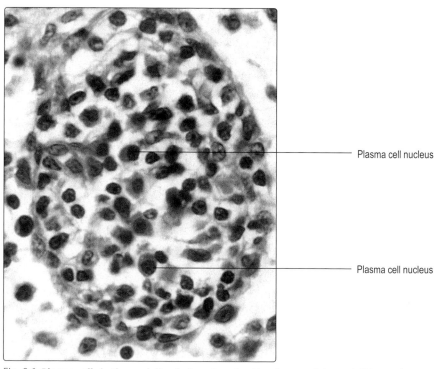

Fig. 8.6 **Plasma cells in the medulla of a lymph node.** The plasma cells have pinkish cytoplasm (reflecting the antibody proteins they contain) and some display an eccentric nucleus. High magnification.

Macrophages

Macrophages are derived from monocytes that have migrated out of blood vessels and many are transient in tissues and organs (e.g. the lungs) and especially in loose connective tissues supporting the parenchymal cells of organs. In certain organs macrophages are present at fixed locations, e.g. as Kupffer cells in the liver (Chapter 12).

Macrophages are able to phagocytose material such as dead cells and bacteria and inert particles, e.g. carbon. Some of the material they ingest (not carbon) is digested in lysosomes and some is presented as antigenic molecules to lymphocytes which then produce an immune response. Macrophages which have taken up inert material, such as carbon, remain in the body and account for the black colour seen in the lungs of many people at post mortem. Macrophage numbers can increase when exposure to antigens increases as monocytes leave peripheral blood and become macrophages.

Dendritic cells (antigen-presenting cells)

Dendritic cells are derived from cells in bone marrow and they are able to present antigens to lymphocytes and this initiates an immune response. Dendritic cells exhibit fine cytoplasmic processes which increase their surface area and hence the area available for antigen binding. They are present in the supporting connective tissue of many parenchymal organs and in lymph nodes. Dendritic cells in the skin are known as Langerhans cells and those in the brain as microglial cells.

The immune system

The immune system may be considered to have two types of response which help to protect the body from foreign molecules, cells and organisms, including viruses, bacteria and parasites.

- *Non-specific responses.* These are carried out by cells such as neutrophils and macrophages which are able to engulf and destroy many microorganisms and molecules. The ability of neutrophils to migrate from blood vessels and find their way rapidly to sites of infection produces an acute inflammatory response which may quickly stop an infection.
- *Specific responses.* The humoral (fluid) and cell-mediated responses carried out, respectively, by B and T

lymphocytes are directed specifically at individual molecules (which may be free or attached to a cell's membrane). Significantly these specific immune responses are associated with the ability of a lymphocyte to 'remember' a molecule it has encountered. At a subsequent meeting with a 'remembered' molecule such lymphocytes rapidly produce an immune response against the molecule and, importantly, also undergo rapid mitotic activity producing more lymphocytes which can also respond to the same molecule. This type of memory response is known as acquired immunity.

Immune cells are produced in the bone marrow, thymus, spleen and lymph nodes. In addition, there are numerous sites, particularly in the respiratory, digestive, urinary and reproductive systems, where lymphocytes are present in large numbers and are able to respond to foreign molecules or microorganisms.

Bone marrow

Bone marrow occupies spaces within bones (Chapter 9). Red and white blood cells and platelets develop in bone marrow in a process known as haematopoiesis. In regions where haematopoiesis occurs the marrow appears red to the unaided eye. With age, many of the haematopoietic regions are replaced by adipose cells which give marrow a yellow colour.

Within bone marrow blood flows in endothelium-lined blood vessels and a reticulin meshwork surrounding the vessels is packed with developing blood cells. Macrophages are associated with the meshwork and they are involved in destroying aged red blood cells. Megakaryocytes are also in the meshwork and they shed fragments of their cytoplasm, as platelets, into adjacent blood vessels. The appearance of bone marrow in sections reveals few details of the structure of the developing blood cells and smears of bone marrow are examined for detailed studies. Megakaryocytes, however, can be identified readily in sectioned material by their large size and multilobed nucleus (Fig. 8.7).

Haematopoiesis

All blood cells arise from one type of stem cell in bone marrow which resembles a small lymphocyte and is described as being pluripotent. These stem cells undergo successive rounds of mitosis and replace themselves and produce cells which are able to differentiate into different types of cell with restricted stem cell ability. After several cycles of mitotic activity the potential to develop into several types of blood cell is restricted and unipotent stem cells develop. Unipotent stem cells are committed to produce one type of blood cell (and replace themselves). Unipotent stem cells are categorised by the type of blood cell they produce. For details of the stages in the formation of erythrocytes, eosinophils, basophils, neutro

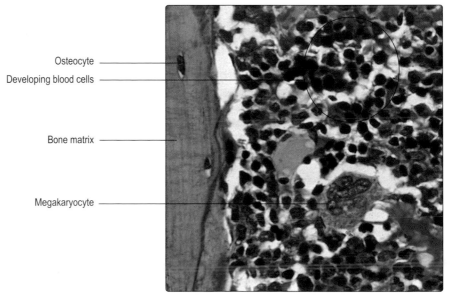

Osteocyte
Developing blood cells

Bone matrix

Megakaryocyte

Fig. 8.7 **Bone marrow.** Megakaryocyte. High magnification.

phils, monocytes, T lymphocytes and B lymphocytes, NK cells and megakaryocytes from stem cells, a more detailed textbook of histology or haematology should be consulted.

The rate of production of new blood cells (and platelets) in the bone marrow normally equals the rate at which each cell type dies. Some blood cells, e.g. neutrophils, live less than a week whereas red blood cells live for about 120 days. Some lymphocytes live 10 or more years. Vast numbers of new blood cells are produced each day (e.g. about 3×10^9 red blood cells/kg body weight are produced each day). Most blood cells leave bone marrow when they are mature by entering blood in vessels in bone marrow. Some cells, such as neutrophils, usually stay in the bone marrow for a few days after they mature and they act as a reservoir of cells that can rapidly enter the circulation and migrate to sites of infection.

Thymus

The thymus is an organ in the mid-line of the upper anterior part of the thorax which is prominent in young children and gradually regresses after puberty. It is covered by a connective tissue capsule and has a fine meshwork which extends throughout the thymus. Unusually, the meshwork is formed by epithelial, not connective tissue, cells. The epithelial mesh supports lymphocytes and two regions, a peripheral cortex and inner medulla, are described. Virtually all of the lymphocytes in the thymus are in direct contact with the epithelial meshwork and the epithelial cells are sometimes referred to as 'nurse' cells.

Lymphocytes are densely packed in the meshwork in the cortex (Fig. 8.8). In the medulla, fewer lymphocytes are present, and they appear in irregular clumps (Fig. 8.8). The most recognisable components of the support meshwork are the epithelial cells which form whorl-like, lamellated structures in the medulla known as Hassall's corpuscles (Fig. 8.8). The function of these corpuscles is not known.

The thymus secretes factors that facilitate its functions. The functions are particularly important in the early stages of life and they are:

- to provide an environment to receive immature T lymphocytes from bone marrow
- to ensure that immature T lymphocytes become

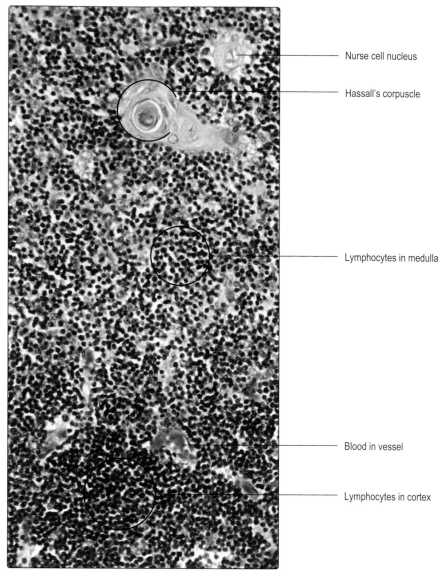

Nurse cell nucleus

Hassall's corpuscle

Lymphocytes in medulla

Blood in vessel

Lymphocytes in cortex

Fig. 8.8 **Thymus, cortex and medulla.** Medium magnification

immunologically competent, i.e. able to produce immune responses to attack foreign molecules, cells and organisms
- to ensure that immature T lymphocytes also become self-tolerant; this process enables T lymphocytes to distinguish 'self' from foreign cells and molecules and thus avoid attacking 'self' body cells and molecules
- to release mature T lymphocytes into circulation.

The processes that produce mature T lymphocytes involve the generation of many new T lymphocytes by mitosis of the T lymphocytes in the cortex of the thymus. Many of these new lymphocytes die; these are thought to be T lymphocytes which are not self-tolerant. Other T lymphocytes move towards the medulla as they mature and become self-tolerant and immunologically com-

petent. The mature T lymphocytes in the medulla are released into blood vessels. They live for many years and many leave the blood vessels and migrate through tissues where they may be triggered into producing immune responses.

Spleen

The spleen lies in the left, upper region of the abdomen. It is the largest lymphoid organ of the body and it has two main functions:

- it monitors circulating blood for foreign material, particularly bacteria, and ensures immune responses develop to such material
- it destroys aged red blood cells, probably when they have become relatively rigid.

The spleen has a connective tissue capsule which is covered by a serosal membrane called the peritoneum (Chapter 3). Connective tissue strands (trabeculae) extend from the capsule into the spleen and these support branches of arterial blood vessels distributing blood through the parenchyma. An intricate network of fine reticulin fibres connected to the trabeculae support the cells in the parenchyma. Two regions known as the red pulp and white pulp form the parenchyma. With the unaided eye the white pulp appears pale and the red pulp appears red: white cells are predominant in white pulp and red blood cells predominant in red pulp.

- *White pulp.* White pulp contains aggregations of lymphocytes packing the reticular meshwork. Many of the lymphocytes in white pulp appear as sheaths around small arteries (arterioles) distributing blood through the spleen. This arrangement is known as a periarteriolar lymphatic sheath (PALS) and is unique to the spleen. These blood vessels are known as central arterioles although they do not always appear to be in the centre of a sheath of lymphocytes (Fig. 8.9). T lymphocytes are predominant in PALS. If lymphocytes in the spleen are responding to foreign material in blood, spherical clusters (follicles) of B lymphocytes appear in the white pulp adjacent to PALS. These are similar in form and function to lymphoid follicles in lymph nodes (see below).

   Some of the blood from central arterioles passes into endothelial-lined blood vessels (also known as sinuses or sinusoids) in the white pulp. These are relatively large spaces where blood moves slowly and blood cells, antigens and particulate matter intermingle. Macrophages attack any microorganisms present and macrophages and other antigen-presenting cells screen particulate matter for foreign antigens and 'present' them to lymphocytes which then mount immune responses.
- *Red pulp.* Red pulp fills the spaces between white pulp. It receives blood that has passed through the central arterioles of the white pulp. The vascular arrangement of the spleen is unusual (in humans) in that some blood and blood cells leak from the sinuses and pass through

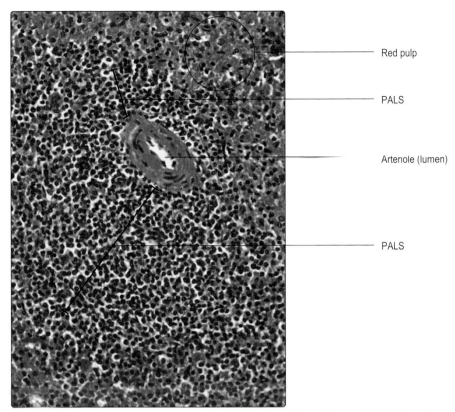

Fig 8.9 **Spleen, red pulp and white pulp with periarteriolar lymphatic sheath (PALS).** Medium magnification

Red pulp

PALS

Arteriole (lumen)

PALS

Clinical note
Autoimmune disorders These are caused by inappropriate immune responses generated against the body's own molecules (which may be free or on cell membranes). In myasthenia gravis, a condition in which muscle weakness and fatigue occurs, autoantibodies are detectable (in most patients) which interfere with synapses at neuromuscular junctions.

---

the meshwork of the red pulp; this is described as an open circulation. Blood in red pulp passes among antigen-presenting cells, macrophages and lymphocytes and then returns into endothelium-lined sinuses. This passage through the red pulp enables immune responses to foreign molecules to develop and ageing red blood cells and platelets to be detected and destroyed. Macrophages ingest and digest the debris from dead cells and useful molecules circulate in blood and are reused. The blood in sinuses drains into venules (small veins) which join together and leave the spleen at the hilum. In addition, a closed circulation may also exist in humans whereby blood does not leave the vessels; instead, it remains in the endothelium-lined sinuses which connect arterioles with venules.

Lymphatic vessels
Lymphatic vessels are lined by endothelial cells and they begin as very small blind-ended tubes in most regions of the body. They serve to drain excess tissue fluid and transmit it through lymph nodes before it returns to peripheral blood in blood vessels (Chapter 10). The fluid in lymph vessels is known as lymph. Valves in lymphatic vessels ensure drainage of lymph is unidirectional, away from an organ or region of the body.

Lymph nodes
Lymph nodes are aggregations of lymphocytes where lymph is monitored for foreign molecules (e.g. in lymph or on bacteria, viruses or tumour cells) and where specific immune responses are generated as a result. Lymph nodes occur in defined anatomical sites where they receive lymph, which is draining

Summary

Blood
- This comprises red and white blood cells and platelets suspended in plasma.
- Blood forms tissue fluid (extracellular fluid) and is able to clot and stop flow from damaged blood vessels.

Red blood cells (erythrocytes)
- These are biconcave discs formed of cytoplasm and a cell membrane (but no nucleus) and are deformable:
  - the cytoplasm consists mainly of haemoglobin, which carries oxygen from the lungs to body tissues
  - red blood cells develop in bone marrow.

White blood cells (leucocytes)
Granulocytes:

- have nuclei with two or more lobes and cytoplasmic granules
- develop in bone marrow, circulate in blood and move into tissues
- are categorised according to the staining characteristics of the granules:
  - neutrophils form 70% of the white cells in blood and phagocytose and kill bacteria
  - eosinophils form about 4% of the white cells in blood and ingest antigen–antibody complexes and kill and ingest parasites
  - basophils form about 1% of the white cells in blood and move into tissue and initiate inflammatory changes.

Agranulocytes:

- have no (or very few) cytoplasmic granules and are categorised according to nuclear shape
  - lymphocytes have spherical nuclei and form about 25% of white blood cells:
    - B lymphocytes respond to antigens by secreting antibodies and T lymphocytes, respond to 'foreign' cells by killing them; NK cells kill 'foreign' cells
  - monocytes have indented nuclei and form about 5% of white blood cells
    - migrate from blood and become macrophages in tissues.

Platelets
- These are small, membrane-bound fragments of cytoplasm that bud off from megakaryocytes in bone marrow. They aid blood clotting.

The immune system
- The immune system defends the body from foreign molecules, cells and organisms.
- It comprises a variety of cells (including white blood cells) in the thymus, spleen, lymph nodes and in mucosal surfaces exposed to the environment.
- It mounts non-specific responses, e.g. phagocytosis by neutrophils, and specific responses, e.g. the humoral response of B lymphocytes and the cell-mediated response of T lymphocytes.
- The immune system also involves mast cells, plasma cells, macrophages and dendritic cells.

Bone marrow
- This comprises a meshwork of reticulin fibres supporting blood vessels and developing red and white blood cells and megakaryocytes which form platelets.

Thymus
- This comprises a meshwork of epithelial cells supporting blood vessels and lymphocytes in an outer cortex densely packed with lymphocytes and an inner medulla where lymphocytes are less densely packed. Hassall's corpuscles are present in the medulla.
- It is particularly active in neonates and regresses with age.
- Lymphocytes leave the thymus and enter the circulation as mature T lymphocytes which recognise self from non-self cells.

Spleen
- This comprises a meshwork of reticulin fibres supporting blood vessels, red blood cells and lymphocytes and various antigen-presenting cells.
- It has red and white pulp regions with sheaths of lymphocytes surrounding arterioles.
- It monitors blood for foreign material and mounts immune responses and destroys aged red blood cells.

Lymphatic vessels and lymph nodes
- Lymphatic vessels drain excess tissue fluid and return the fluid as lymph via lymph nodes to blood vessels.
- Lymph nodes have an outer cortex and inner medulla region and receive lymph from numerous afferent lymph vessels.
- In the cortex, spherical aggregations (follicles) of lymphocytes are numerous.
- Lymph percolates through the cortex and lymphocytes may mount immune responses to foreign molecules or cells in lymph.
- Lymph and cells then pass into the medulla where there are cords of immune cells, which may include plasma cells, and sinuses transporting the lymph.
- A single efferent duct drains lymph from the medulla, and eventually all lymph drains into the cardiovascular circulation.

Chapter 9
Bone and cartilage

Bone and cartilage are derived from the mesoderm layer of the embryo and are specialised forms of connective tissue. Together with other connective tissue and skeletal muscle they constitute the musculoskeletal system. The musculoskeletal system is involved in producing movement and stability of the body by transmitting and resisting forces produced by, for instance, muscle contraction and gravity. Common features of bone and cartilage are that they contain connective tissue fibres and ground substance, forming an extracellular matrix which is relatively rigid compared with the rest of the body and is able to resist mechanical stress. In the extracellular matrix, collagen fibres are important in resisting tensile forces and elastin fibres are capable of deformation under stretching forces (and they recoil when the force is reduced).

Cartilage

Cartilage has cellular and non-cellular components. Cartilage cells (chondrocytes) lie in spaces, known as lacunae, surrounded by cartilage matrix (the non-cellular component) (Fig. 9.1). The matrix is produced by cartilage cells and it is a semi-solid material composed of ground substance comprising large molecules (e.g. glycosaminoglycans and proteoglycans), water and connective tissue fibres. Cartilage in many regions is surrounded by a thin layer of connective tissue known as the perichondrium, which is composed mainly of fibroblasts (Fig. 9.1). However, there are sites where perichondrium is not adjacent to cartilage, e.g. on the articulating surfaces of bone (Fig. 9.2). Blood capillaries are not present in cartilage and the oxygen and nutrients required by chondrocytes diffuse through the matrix from nearby capillaries in the perichondrium.

There are three types of cartilage defined by the major type of fibre present:

- *hyaline cartilage* contains mainly type II collagen fibres and is the most abundant type of cartilage in the body
- *elastic cartilage* contains type II collagen and elastin fibres
- *fibrocartilage* contains type I collagen fibres.

Hyaline cartilage
Hyaline cartilage is present in a wide range of locations and is important in resisting forces and in supporting soft tissues. It forms the articulating surfaces of bones in synovial joints (Fig. 9.2), where it provides a smooth, friction-free surface at which movements occur, and it acts as a shock absorber. Hyaline cartilage also aids respiration by providing rigidity in the larynx, trachea and bronchi, thus ensuring their patency during inspiration (Chapter 11). It is also present at the anterior ends of ribs where movements of the rib cage occur during respiration. In the embryo, hyaline cartilage forms a temporary skeleton which eventually is largely replaced by bone (see below).

There are two cell types in hyaline cartilage: chondroblasts and chondrocytes. Chondroblasts are able to undergo mitosis and secrete extracellular cartilage matrix. They are very active metabolically and may appear in small clusters. Such clusters (Fig. 9.2) contain new cells produced by mitosis from one initial cell in the region. Chondrocytes are the mature form of chondroblasts

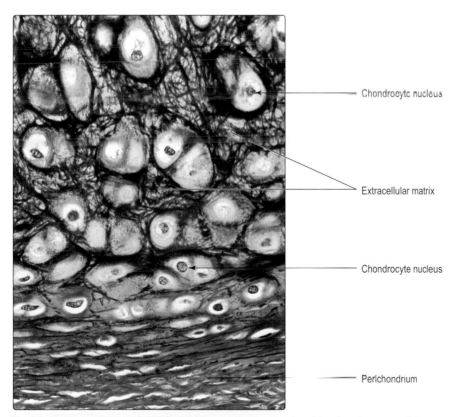

Fig. 9.1 **Elastic cartilage and perichondrium, epiglottis.** The size of the chondrocytes, and the lacunae they occupy, varies. Elastin fibres appear as dark strands in the extracellular matrix. Special stain. High magnification.

Chondrocyte nucleus

Extracellular matrix

Chondrocyte nucleus

Perichondrium

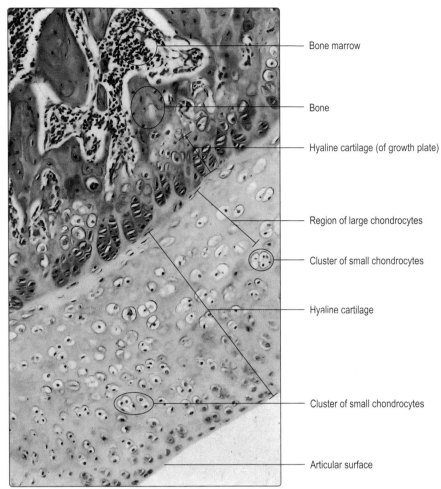

Bone marrow

Bone

Hyaline cartilage (of growth plate)

Region of large chondrocytes

Cluster of small chondrocytes

Hyaline cartilage

Cluster of small chondrocytes

Articular surface

Fig. 9.2 **Hyaline cartilage of an articular surface of bone from a synovial joint.** Medium magnification.

and are no longer able to undergo mitosis but can still secrete and modify cartilage matrix. The main chemical components of hyaline cartilage matrix are proteoglycans, glycosaminoglycans and hyaluronic acid, which all attract water molecules. This composition allows hyaline cartilage to resist compressive forces and act as a shock absorber. The type of collagen fibres (type II) and their orientation in hyaline cartilage are important in resisting mechanical forces. The appearance of hyaline cartilage is described as 'glassy' and the collagen fibres are not apparent in routine histological preparations. With age, chondrocytes and the lacunae they occupy enlarge (Fig. 9.2) and calcium salts may be deposited in the matrix. These changes may alter the mechanical properties of the cartilage.

Growth in hyaline cartilage occurs by two modes: interstitial and appositional growth. Interstitial growth (growth from within) occurs mainly in the early stage of cartilage development. In interstitial growth, cartilage cells in lacunae undergo mitosis, produce matrix and separate from one another; the matrix occupies

increasingly larger regions between the cells. Appositional growth occurs at the periphery of clusters of cartilage cells, adjacent to the perichondrium. Fibroblasts in the innermost part of the perichondrium are specialised and known as chondrogenic cells as they can become chondroblasts and secrete cartilage matrix. Most cartilage in the body grows by appositional growth. However, there are exceptions. For example, articular cartilage is not invested by perichondrium (Fig. 9.2) and grows only by interstitial growth. Furthermore, growth of long bones, which occurs up to the age of about 20 years, also occurs via interstitial growth of cartilage (see below).

Elastic cartilage

There are similarities between the structure and mode of growth of hyaline and elastic cartilage. However, chondrocytes in elastic cartilage are larger than those in hyaline cartilage and the volume of matrix is less. The matrix of elastic cartilage contains type II collagen fibres, but in addition it has an abundance of elastin fibres which confers on the cartilage a

degree of deformability and recoil. The elastin fibres may be readily displayed using special stains (Fig. 9.1). Elastic cartilage is present in, for example, the epiglottis and the external ear.

Fibrocartilage

Fibrocartilage is present in the secondary cartilaginous joints of the body, e.g. in intervertebral discs (Fig. 9.3). Fibrocartilage is not invested by perichondrium and in general it is less rigid than hyaline cartilage. The chondrocytes in fibrocartilage often appear oriented along the lines of stress on the cartilage and there are intervening layers of collagen fibres (type I). Fibrocartilage provides resistance to mechanical forces and sometimes is also present in the dense, regular connective tissue in tendons and ligaments.

Bone

Bone plays a vital physical role in protecting delicate underlying body structures, e.g. the heart and brain. Collectively, bones form the jointed skeleton of the body and, in conjunction with the attachment sites of skeletal muscles and tendons, bones act as levers and enable movements to occur. Although bone is hard and apparently inert, it is able to remodel in response to changes, e.g. in the stresses acting upon it, particularly during growth, exercise and after fracture. In addition, calcium in bone acts as a store for use by the rest of the body if calcium uptake in the diet is inadequate. Bone also provides the framework for body shape (along with fat and muscle) and spaces in bones, filled with bone marrow, are sites where blood cell formation (haematopoiesis) occurs (Chapter 8).

Bone consists of several types of bone cell and associated bone matrix. Most bone cells in adults are osteocytes and they lie in lacunae embedded in extracellular bone matrix. Although bone matrix resembles cartilage matrix (Fig. 9.4) it has organic and inorganic components. The organic components of bone matrix include type I collagen fibres, proteoglycans and glycosaminoglycans. The inorganic component of bone matrix consists largely of calcium hydroxyapatite $(Ca_{10}(PO_4)_6(OH)_2)$. The hydroxyapatite is deposited alongside the collagen fibres and this produces the rigid hardness of bone. In comparison with cartilage matrix, the composition of bone matrix restricts the diffusion of gases, nutrients and waste molecules.

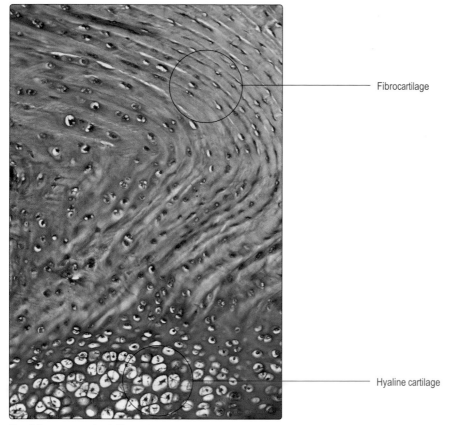

Fibrocartilage

Hyaline cartilage

Fig. 9.3 **Intervertebral disc.** Fibrocartilage and hyaline cartilage. Special stain. Medium magnification.

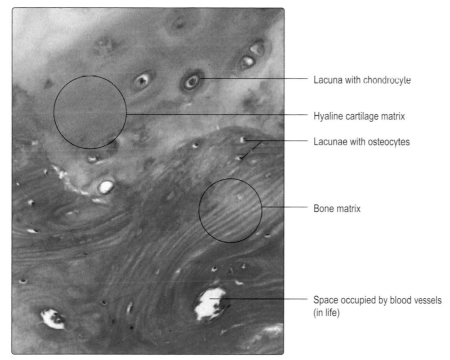

Lacuna with chondrocyte

Hyaline cartilage matrix

Lacunae with osteocytes

Bone matrix

Space occupied by blood vessels (in life)

Fig. 9.4 **Bone and hyaline cartilage.** Only the nuclei of osteocytes and chondrocytes are apparent (in their lacunae) at this magnification. In some regions, the regular arrangement of bone matrix helps distinguish it from the smooth 'glassy' appearance of hyaline cartilage matrix. Low magnification.

However, bone matrix is permeated by small blood vessels (capillaries), an arrangement that ensures osteocytes receive sufficient oxygen and nutrients.

Individual bones are covered by a thin layer of connective tissue (the periosteum) except at some joint surfaces, e.g. in synovial joints the ends of the bones are covered by hyaline cartilage (Fig. 9.2). Periosteum contains collagen fibres, small blood vessels and fibroblasts, which can differentiate and become bone-forming cells. Importantly, collagen fibres surrounding many skeletal muscle cells and those in tendons and ligaments are anchored to periosteum and pass through into the bone matrix as Sharpey's fibres. Such collagen fibres transfer forces from muscles, tendons and ligaments to bones.

There are four major cell types in bone: osteoprogenitor cells, osteoblasts, osteocytes and osteoclasts.

■ *Osteoprogenitor cells* are fibroblast-like cells in the inner layer of the periosteum adjacent to the surface of bone; they function as stem cells. In actively growing bone or after fracture they undergo mitosis. Some offspring cells differentiate into osteoblasts whilst others remain as osteoprogenitor cells.

■ *Osteoblasts* (Fig. 9.5) are present at the surface of bone matrix (and the surface of hyaline cartilage matrix in growing bones; see below). Their appearance depends on their level of activity in synthesising new matrix: inactive osteoblasts have little cytoplasm but active ones may appear polygonal or cuboidal in shape. Active osteoblasts have an abundance of rough endoplasmic reticulum in their cytoplasm, reflecting their activity in secreting the organic components of bone matrix. Newly formed bone matrix, deposited onto the surface of existing matrix, does not contain calcium salts and is known as osteoid. Rapidly, osteoid becomes mineralised by the addition of calcium salts and this forms bone matrix. Osteoblasts are essential in this calcification process, which confers rigidity on bone.

In contrast to the growth of cartilage, bone growth occurs only by the appositional method of adding matrix onto the surface of existing matrix. Once osteoblasts are surrounded by bone matrix they become osteocytes and do not

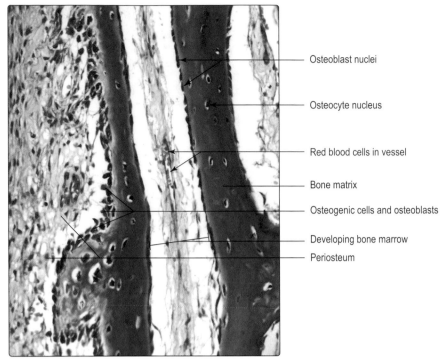

Fig. 9.5 **Bone and periosteum.** The cells on the surface of bone adjacent to the periosteum include osteogenic cells and osteoblasts but distinguishing them at this magnification is not possible. Medium magnification.

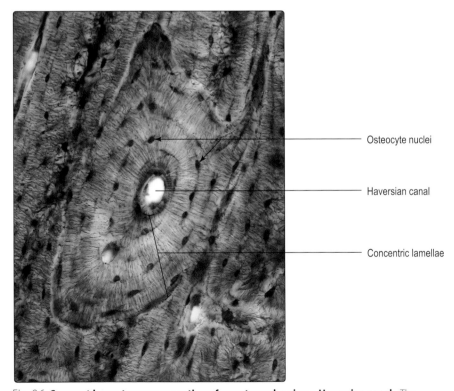

Fig. 9.6 **Compact bone, transverse section of an osteon showing a Haversian canal.** The canaliculi (spaces occupied by cytoplasmic processes of osteocytes) appear as very fine dark strands radiating from the Haversian canal to osteocytes. Only the nuclei of osteocytes are clearly seen. Special stain. High magnification.

undergo mitosis; thus, interstitial growth does not occur.

- *Osteocytes* are mature bone cells and they are located in lacunae surrounded by bone matrix (Figs 9.4 and 9.5). They are relatively inactive cells. Long cytoplasmic processes extend from osteocytes and pass in channels (canaliculi) in bone matrix (Fig. 9.6). Through these cytoplasmic processes osteocytes are able to exchange gases and molecules with blood in nearby capillaries in bone matrix (see below). Osteocytes are involved in metabolic processes which help maintain bone matrix.
- *Osteoclasts* are involved in the remodelling of bone such as that occurring during growth, development and fracture repair. Unlike other bone cells which are derived from fibroblast-like cells, osteoclasts are derived from blood monocytes. Osteoclasts are large, multinucleated cells (Fig. 9.7) and they lie on the surface of bone matrix, sometimes occupying small depressions known as Howship's lacunae. Osteoclasts secrete enzymes onto the bone matrix that digest the matrix releasing ions and small molecules, e.g. calcium and phosphate ions and amino acids. The released small molecules enter blood vessels, circulate and are available for use elsewhere in the body.

The activity of osteoclasts is under the control of two hormones (Chapter 14) that ensure circulating blood levels of calcium are regulated. Parathyroid hormone stimulates osteoclasts to resorb bone and this raises blood calcium. Osteoclast activity is inhibited by calcitonin from the parafollicular cells of the thyroid gland and this lowers blood calcium.

Types of bone

Most bones in the body contain compact (dense) and cancellous (spongy) bone. Compact bone is very dense compared with cancellous bone (Fig. 9.8). In a typical adult long bone, e.g. the humerus, compact bone forms an outer collar along the shaft (diaphysis), whereas cancellous bone constitutes the less dense interior. Cancellous bone forms most of the ends of long bones (the epiphyses) in adults although compact bone may form a thin rim. (Hyaline cartilage is also a component of epiphyses of bones involved in synovial joints and it covers

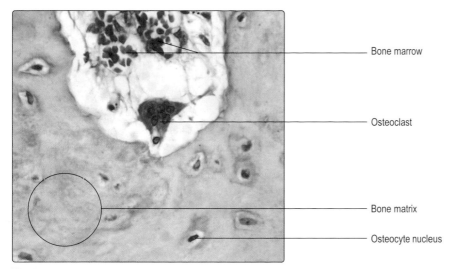

Bone marrow

Osteoclast

Bone matrix

Osteocyte nucleus

Fig. 9.7 **Osteoclast.** High magnification.

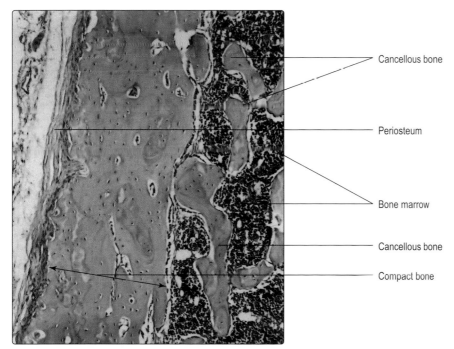

Cancellous bone

Periosteum

Bone marrow

Cancellous bone

Compact bone

Fig. 9.8 **Compact and cancellous bone and bone marrow.** Low magnification.

the joint surface.) Spaces within cancellous bone (Fig. 9.8) are filled by bone marrow, which is involved in blood cell formation, and fat cells; the number of fat cells increases with age.

Compact bone is based on an arrangement of bone cells and matrix known as the Haversian system. This arrangement consists of many thin layers (lamellae) of bone (Fig. 9.6) arranged concentrically as cylinders which lie along the length of the shaft of long bones. This arrangement gives maximal resistance to forces acting along the bone and is particularly important in resisting compression due to weight bearing. Osteocytes, in lacunae, are embedded within the lamellae and lie in concentric circles which are apparent if the cylinders are sectioned across their length, i.e. transversely (Figs 9.6 and 9.9). At the centre of each cylinder of lamellae are small blood and lymphatic vessels and nerves in a space known as a Haversian canal (Figs 9.6 and 9.9). Cytoplasmic processes of osteocytes extend through very small channels (canaliculi) in the bone matrix (Fig. 9.6) and via this route exchange gases and molecules with blood in vessels in a nearby Haversian canal. The whole unit of a Haversian canal plus lamellae is known as an osteon. Although Haversian systems have such a highly regular arrangement of osteons, in many regions the cylinders are packed together with irregular lamellae of bone (Fig. 9.9). The regularity of the cylinders of osteons is also apparent when they are sectioned along their length (Fig. 9.10). In addition, canals (Volkmann's) carry vessels and nerves perpendicular to Haversian canals. The presence of blood vessels in bone matrix ensures all osteocytes have adequate oxygen and nutrients, without which they die and the bone matrix degenerates.

Cancellous bone consists of thin spicules (trabeculae) of bone that project as a meshwork from compact bone (Fig. 9.8). This type of bone has a random lamellar structure with osteocytes located in lacunae but it does not have Haversian or Volkmann's canals. The osteocytes are nourished via diffusion from blood vessels in the marrow.

Bone formation and growth

Bone formation (ossification) and growth of bones begins in utero and continues up to the age of 20 or so. After this time, ossification and bone growth stops but the components of matrix are gradually removed and/or replaced throughout life. In addition, at any stage,

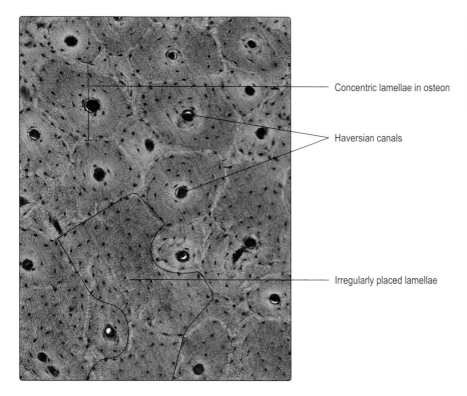

Concentric lamellae in osteon

Haversian canals

Irregularly placed lamellae

Fig. 9.9 **Compact bone, transverse section of osteons showing their Haversian canals.** Nuclei of osteocytes appear as small dark dots; some lie in concentric circles formed by lamellae of bone. A black line surrounds some irregularly placed lamellae. Special stain. Medium magnification.

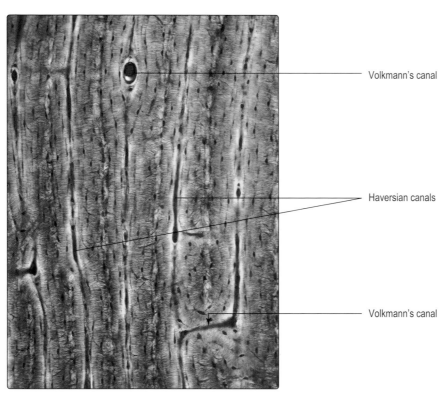

Volkmann's canal

Haversian canals

Volkmann's canal

Fig. 9.10 **Compact bone, longitudinal section of osteons.** Nuclei of osteocytes appear as small dark dots in rows formed by lamellae of bone. Special stain. Medium magnification.

the shape of bones may be remodelled in response to various factors including dietary changes, strenuous exercise or physical damage. Bone formation and growth occurs by two methods: intramembranous and endochondral ossification.

Intramembranous ossification
This type of bone formation and growth is associated only with flat bones, such as the clavicle and some bones in the skull. In regions where these bones develop, some fibroblast-like cells (osteoprogenitor cells) derived from mesoderm of the embryo differentiate into osteoblasts which then secrete an irregular framework of bone matrix. Growth occurs as further fibroblast-like cells on the surface of the developing bone differentiate and become osteoblasts which then add bone matrix onto the existing matrix, i.e. by appositional growth.

Endochondral ossification
The majority of bones in the skeletal system are formed, and grow, by endochondral ossification. In this process a 'model' of hyaline cartilage, comprising chondrocytes and cartilage matrix in the shape of the adult bone, develops first (Fig. 9.11). The cartilage model grows and gradually bone matrix and bone cells replace the cartilage in the diaphysis. In growing long bones the diaphysis is separated from each epiphysis by an

epiphyseal growth plate (EGP) of cartilage. This is the region where many bones grow in length until adulthood.

There are several stages in endochondral ossification.

1. Hyaline cartilage model forms (Fig. 9.11).
   - Some bones (e.g. the femur) begin to form in utero at about 6 weeks (in humans).
   - Appositional and interstitial growth occurs in the cartilage model and shape develops.
   - Chondrocytes in the centre of the model increase in size.
   - Calcium salts are deposited in the matrix around the older chondrocytes, which eventually die (see below).
2. Collar of bone forms (Fig. 9.12).
   - Osteogenic cells and blood vessels develop in the perichondrium.
   - The osteogenic cells become osteoblasts which form a collar of bone (bone cells and matrix) around the diaphysis. This is described as a primary ossification centre.
   - The perichondrium in the region of the bone becomes periosteum.
3. Invasion of the bone collar occurs (Fig. 9.13).
   - Cells in the periosteum invade the collar of bone forming a 'periosteal bud'.
   - The invasion brings osteogenic cells (and cells which form red and white blood cells and blood vessels) into the diaphysis.
4. The large old chondrocytes die and disappear; bone and bone marrow form (Figs 9.13 and 9.14).
   - Chondrocytes die and leave a loose meshwork of cartilage matrix.
   - The invading cells from the periosteal bud enter the spaces left in old, calcified cartilage matrix.
   - Osteoblasts (developed from the invading osteogenic cells) secrete bone matrix onto the calcified cartilage matrix.
   - Osteoblasts surrounded by bone matrix become osteocytes (Fig. 9.15).
   - Bone marrow forms from the invading cells as red and white blood cells and blood vessels develop.
5. Ossification extends.
   - Osteoblasts continue to deposit bone matrix onto cartilage matrix at each end of the diaphysis.

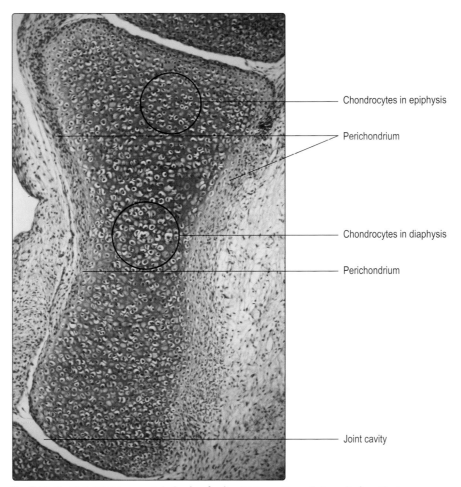

Fig. 9.11 **Hyaline cartilage model of a developing bone sectioned along its length.** Low magnification.

Chondrocytes in epiphysis
Perichondrium
Chondrocytes in diaphysis
Perichondrium
Joint cavity

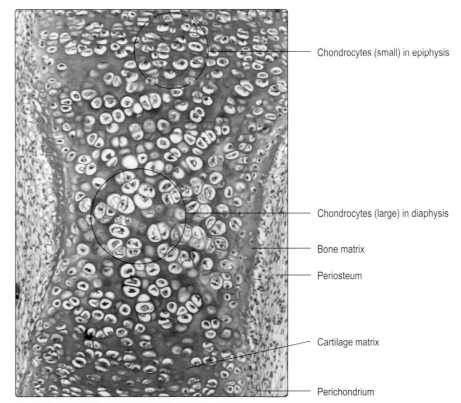

Fig. 9.12 **Bone collar around diaphysis of a developing bone (sectioned along its length).** The osteocytes in the bone matrix can be distinguished by their nuclei which appear as small dots in the pink-stained matrix. Medium magnification.

Chondrocytes (small) in epiphysis
Chondrocytes (large) in diaphysis
Bone matrix
Periosteum
Cartilage matrix
Perichondrium

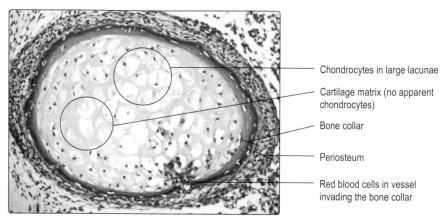

Chondrocytes in large lacunae

Cartilage matrix (no apparent chondrocytes)

Bone collar

Periosteum

Red blood cells in vessel invading the bone collar

Fig. 9.13 **Invasion of bone collar (sectioned across the length of the bone).** The invasion involves blood in vessels, osteogenic cells and stem cells capable of forming blood cells. Only red cells can be distinguished in this micrograph. Medium magnification.

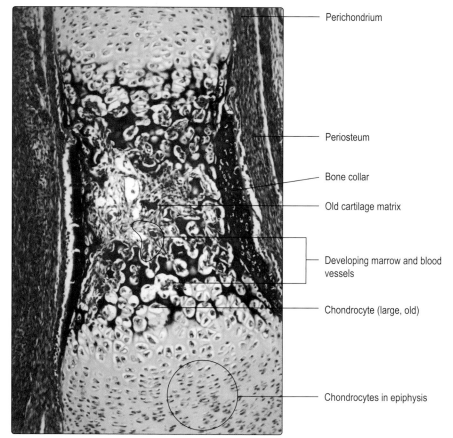

Perichondrium

Periosteum

Bone collar

Old cartilage matrix

Developing marrow and blood vessels

Chondrocyte (large, old)

Chondrocytes in epiphysis

Fig. 9.14 **Chondrocyte loss, bone and bone marrow formation.** Chondrocytes have died and disappeared from the centre of the diaphysis and only a few remnants of cartilage matrix remain there. Low magnification.

- Chondrocytes remain as an EGP (Fig. 9.16) at each end of a diaphysis for several years. Chondrocytes produced by mitosis in these plates are responsible for the growth in length of bones until adulthood.

Growth in length of bone at epiphyseal plates

EGPs have several zones involved in ensuring each diaphysis grows in length. Each zone merges with adjacent zones (Fig. 9.15 and 9.16).

- *Zone of reserve cartilage.* This is the hyaline cartilage connecting each EGP to the adjacent epiphysis.
- *Zone of proliferation.* Chondrocytes proliferate rapidly and new chondrocytes extend as columns of cells parallel to the long axis of the bone and away from the epiphysis. This is interstitial growth. Older chondrocytes in the columns, those farthest from the reserve zone, begin to secrete cartilage matrix. By forming these new cells and matrix in columns, the length of the diaphysis is extended and a framework is formed on which bone is later deposited.
- *Zone of hypertrophy.* With increasing age chondrocytes enlarge.
- *Zone of calcification and chondrocyte death.* Calcium salts are deposited in the cartilage matrix and the oldest chondrocytes die, probably due to programmed cell death (apoptosis).
- *Zone of ossification.* Osteoprogenitor cells migrate from the diaphysis and become osteoblasts as they secrete bone matrix onto the surface of the calcified cartilage matrix. This process extends the length of the bone of the diaphysis. Calcium salts are then deposited into the bone matrix and some osteoblasts become surrounded by bone matrix and become osteocytes (Fig. 9.15).

Growth in width of bone

Circumferential growth of each diaphysis occurs as osteoprogenitor cells in the periosteum become osteoblasts and lay bone matrix on the outer surface of the shaft (appositional growth). At the same time osteoclasts remove bone from the inner surface of the shaft. As a result the width of the outer rim of compact bone is adjusted and does not become thicker as the overall width of the bone increases. Gradually, the adult distribution of cancellous and dense bone develops.

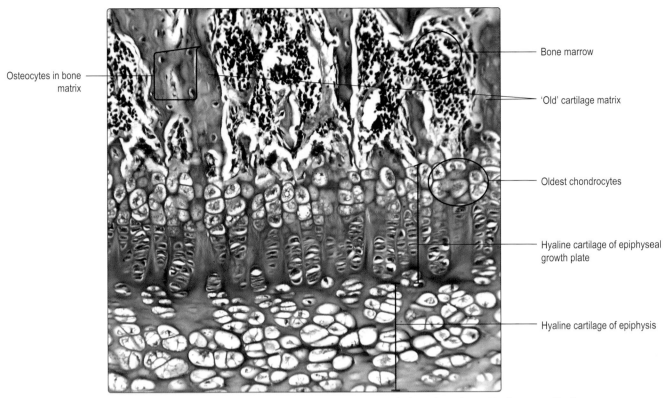

Osteocytes in bone matrix

Bone marrow

'Old' cartilage matrix

Oldest chondrocytes

Hyaline cartilage of epiphyseal growth plate

Hyaline cartilage of epiphysis

Fig. 9.15 **Epiphyseal growth plate.** See text for details of the processes occurring in growth plates. Special stain. Medium magnification.

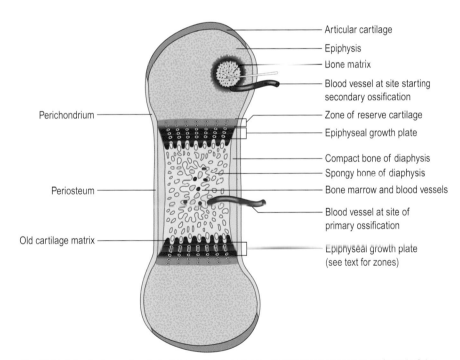

Articular cartilage
Epiphysis
Bone matrix
Blood vessel at site starting secondary ossification
Zone of reserve cartilage
Epiphyseal growth plate
Compact bone of diaphysis
Spongy bone of diaphysis
Bone marrow and blood vessels
Blood vessel at site of primary ossification
Epiphyseal growth plate (see text for zones)

Perichondrium

Periosteum

Old cartilage matrix

Fig. 9.16 **A typical growing long bone.** Epiphyseal growth plates are present at each end of the diaphysis. In one epiphysis a secondary ossification centre has started to replace the hyaline cartilage with bone.

Remodelling of bone

There is considerable remodelling of the shaft of long bones through resorption of matrix and deposition of new bone matrix. The regions where bone matrix is initially deposited on cartilage matrix are digested by osteoclasts at the same time as new bone is added to existing bone matrix.

Growth of epiphyses and cessation of growth

Interstitial growth of cartilage, and appositional growth (in regions adjacent to perichondrium), increases the volume of each epiphysis. Just after birth, small regions develop where blood vessels and osteogenic cells invade some epiphyses, a process described as secondary ossification (Fig. 9.16). Gradually, over the next 20 years or so, bone and bone marrow replace the hyaline cartilage of epiphyses, except at surfaces involved in synovial joints where hyaline cartilage remains.

Epiphyses fuse with their diaphysis as bone replaces the hyaline cartilage of the growth plates. The time at which this ossification occurs differs between different bones in the body. These times are relatively constant between individuals.

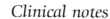

Clinical notes

Osteoporosis This condition results from a decreased level of calcium in bones. Age-related loss of bone mineral density occurs in all persons to an extent. In women especially, there is increased activity of osteoclasts after the menopause as oestrogen levels decrease due to the loss of secretion of these hormones from the ovaries. The affected bones are often fractured with minimal force. Oestrogen therapy, and high intake of calcium, helps to slow the disease progression.

Genetic disorders These may affect epiphyseal growth plates and result in individuals shorter or taller than normal. (Epiphyseal growth plates and adult height may also be abnormal as a result of abnormal levels of growth hormone secreted by the pituitary gland.)

Osteoarthritis and rheumatoid arthritis These inflammatory processes that occur in cartilage are common. Osteoarthritis affects the hyaline cartilage covering the ends of articulating bones, particularly affecting weight-bearing joints such as knees, hips and ankles. In this disease the cartilage slowly degenerates with age, with underlying damage affecting the bone. In contrast, rheumatoid arthritis is a systemic autoimmune disease that affects other organs and tissues as well as joints. Because of its widespread effects, rheumatoid arthritis is much more difficult to treat. Rheumatoid arthritis, in contrast to osteoarthritis, may affect young people and may pursue a much more aggressive course.

Summary

Bone and cartilage

- These are connective tissues with relatively rigid extracellular matrix containing collagen fibres and large molecules containing carbohydrates. Bone is more rigid than cartilage and has extensive deposits of calcium salts in the extracellular matrix.
- Mature cartilage and bone cells (respectively, chondrocytes and osteocytes) occupy spaces (lacunae) in the matrix.
- Osteocytes in many regions are nourished by a network of capillaries in Haversian canals.

Cartilage

- This occurs in three types:
  - hyaline cartilage forms the smooth articulating surfaces of many bones and has a major role in skeletal development
  - elastic cartilage has a matrix containing elastin and collagen and is able to recoil after being deformed
  - fibrous cartilage provides resistance to mechanical forces.
- Cartilage grows by appositional and interstitial growth.

Bone

- Bone protects many organs and provides firm attachments for muscles and tendons which allows movements to occur.
- It may be described as compact (dense) or cancellous (spongy):
  - in compact bone the matrix comprises cylinders of lamellae of bone around blood vessels in a Haversian canal
  - in cancellous bone thin trabeculae of bone matrix form a meshwork.
- It begins to develop in utero as a hyaline cartilage model and becomes bone by endochondral ossification. (A few bones form directly by intramembranous ossification.)
- In endochondral ossification the hyaline cartilage model grows by interstitial and appositional growth.
- The cartilage is replaced as chondrocytes die and osteogenic cells become osteoblasts which deposit bone matrix on old cartilage matrix.
- Up to about 20 years of age cartilage persists in some bones as an epiphyseal growth plate (EGP) between the diaphysis and an epiphysis. Growth in the length of bones is a result of cartilage cells proliferating in EGPs and bone matrix being deposited on old cartilage matrix.
- Osteoclasts digest bone and are involved in remodelling during growth, development and repair.

Chapter 10
The circulatory system

The circulatory system consists of the heart and the vessels (tubes) which carry blood or lymph. The heart provides a force that moves blood in the vessels of the cardiovascular system. This part of the circulatory system, the cardiovascular system, ensures blood, carrying oxygen, carbon dioxide, various nutrients, metabolites, hormones and blood cells, is conveyed to, through and from the tissues and organs of the body.

Part of the circulatory system comprises lymphatic vessels which drain some of the extracellular fluid from all regions of the body except the central nervous system. The fluid in lymphatic vessels is known as lymph. It is similar to plasma but does not transport red cells. Lymph is an important means of transporting immune cells, particularly lymphocytes, and lymph vessels carry lymph into and out of lymph nodes (Chapter 8). Lymphatic vessels in the gastrointestinal system also transport lipids absorbed from the gut (Chapter

12). Lymph eventually drains into larger lymph vessels which in turn drain into the blood vessels of the cardiovascular system returning blood to the heart.

Cardiovascular system

The heart is an organ which consists of two muscular pumps that work in synchrony. The two pumps are attached side by side but blood, in adults, does not pass directly between the two sides. The heart develops (in utero) from a single tube which duplicates and twists and only takes on the adult structure and the physical separation of the two sides shortly after birth (see Mitchell B, Sharma R. *Embryology: An Illustrated Colour Text.* Elsevier: 2004).

Arteries are vessels which carry blood away from the heart whilst vessels carrying blood to the heart are veins (Fig. 10.1). Blood is carried between arteries and veins in small vessels, arterioles, capillaries and venules. Veins deliver

deoxygenated blood to the right side of the heart, which pumps it into pulmonary arteries and on to the lungs. In the lungs, the deoxygenated blood passes into capillaries and there it becomes oxygenated. The oxygenated blood returns to the left side of the heart via pulmonary veins. This flow of blood between heart and lungs is known as the pulmonary circulation. Simultaneously, the left side of the heart pumps oxygenated blood into the aorta (the largest artery) from where it is distributed around the whole body. Arterial blood passes through progressively branching and narrowing arterial vessels and eventually through the narrowest vessels, the capillaries. It is from capillaries that oxygen diffuses into surrounding tissues and blood becomes deoxygenated. Capillaries drain into venules and these in turn drain into veins which return the deoxygenated blood to the right side of the heart. This flow of blood around the body is described as the systemic circulation.

In some regions of the body, e.g. the liver (Fig. 10.1), in addition to arterial blood delivering oxygenated blood to capillaries, other blood enters the capillaries from a vein. In the case of the liver, capillaries draining blood from the gut join together and drain into the hepatic portal vein. This portal vein, carrying nutrients absorbed from the gut, supplies blood to capillaries in the liver. This arrangement of vessels involving two sets of capillaries joined by a vein is described as a portal circulation.

Heart

Each side of the heart has two compartments: an atrium and a ventricle (Fig. 10.2). The left atrium receives blood from the lungs in four pulmonary veins and the right atrium receives blood from the rest of the body via the superior and inferior vena cavea. The atria simultaneously contract and pump blood into the paired ventricles. The ventricles then pump the blood into

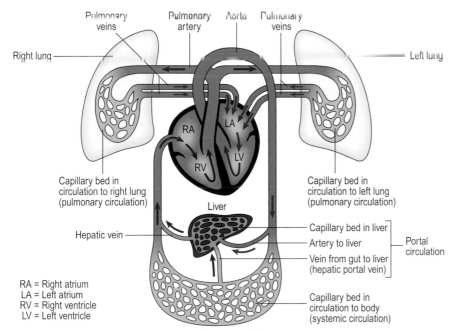

RA = Right atrium
LA = Left atrium
RV = Right ventricle
LV = Left ventricle

Fig. 10.1 **The cardiovascular components (heart and the systemic, pulmonary and portal circulations) of the circulatory system.** Arrows indicate the direction of flow of oxygenated blood (red) and deoxygenated blood (blue).

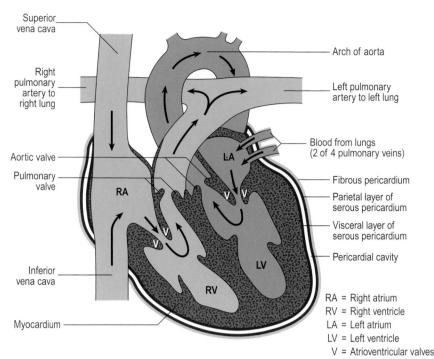

Fig. 10.2 **The internal structure of the heart, the major blood vessels and the pericardium.** Arrows indicate the direction of flow of blood. V, valves between atria and ventricles.

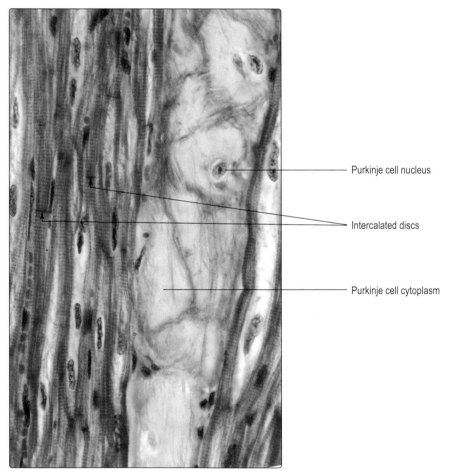

Fig. 10.3 **Heart myocardium with cardiac muscle and Purkinje cells.** Transverse striations are apparent in cardiac muscle cells sectioned along their length as lighter and darker regions of pink-stained sarcoplasm. Intercalated discs appear as darker, wider, pink-stained bands. The glycogen packing the cytoplasm of Purkinje cells is palely stained as glycogen does not react well with the stain used. Connective tissue is stained green. Special stain. High magnification.

either the systemic circulation (left ventricle) or the pulmonary circulation (right ventricle). Valves between each atrium and its ventricle ensure that blood does not flow back into the atria when the ventricles contract. Other valves prevent back flow of blood from the arteries to the ventricles when the ventricles relax. The contraction of heart muscle is regulated by the autonomic nervous system, though heart muscle cells have an intrinsic ability to contract.

The wall of the heart is described as having three layers: the myocardium is the middle and thickest layer, the inner layer is the endocardium and the outer layer is the epicardium. In addition, connective tissue is an important component which ensures normal heart contraction occurs.

- *Myocardium.* The myocardium forms the majority of the wall of the heart: it consists mainly of cardiac muscle cells supported by sparse, fibrous connective tissue. If these muscle cells are sectioned along their length, transverse striations are apparent (Fig. 10.3), reflecting the arrangement of myofilaments in the sarcoplasm of the cells (Chapter 5). Specialised junctions (intercalated discs) attach cells together in series and may be apparent as transverse lines (Fig. 10.3). Although heart muscle cells have an intrinsic ability to contract, sympathetic and parasympathetic nerves are able, respectively, to increase and decrease the rate at which the heart beats. The contraction of cardiac muscle cells is coordinated by specialised cells in several regions of the heart and by communication, via intercalated discs, between individual muscle cells. One specialised cell type, the Purkinje cell, conducts electrical impulses to specific parts of the myocardium so that atria and ventricles contract at appropriate times and blood flows smoothly from atria to ventricles then into the arteries. Purkinje cells are distinguished by their rounded shape (Fig. 10.3) and they have a high content of glycogen.
- *Endocardium.* This lines the myocardium. It is made up of a surface layer of squamous epithelial cells, their basement membrane and a sparse layer of connective tissue attaching the endocardium to the myocardium. The epithelial cells of

the endocardium are similar to, and continuous with, the endothelial cells lining the blood vessels carrying blood to and from the heart.

- *Epicardium*. The epicardium covers the heart and comprises a single layer of squamous epithelial cells, their basement membrane and loose connective tissue which attaches it to the underlying myocardium. Coronary blood vessels supply blood to the heart and lie in the epicardium, in which fat cells may be present in large numbers (Fig. 10.4).

The epicardium is part of a closed sac, the pericardium, which enfolds the heart (Fig. 10.2). It is the inner, visceral layer of the pericardium and is continuous with the outer parietal layer. Each of these two layers is composed of a squamous epithelium, basement membrane and supporting connective tissue and they enclose a potential space, the pericardial cavity. The secretion of minute amounts of fluid into the pericardial cavity by the lining of squamous epithelial cells ensures a relatively friction-free zone against which the heart can move and beat without damaging adjacent cells.

Connective tissue of the heart

Some connective tissue of the heart is condensed and described as a fibrous skeleton. It is a complex arrangement of dense collagen between the atria and ventricles, and around the orifices of the arteries taking blood from the heart (Fig. 10.4). The connective tissue ensures electrical discontinuity between the myocardium of the atria and ventricles except via the specialised conducting tissue; this is essential for the normal rhythm of heart contraction. In addition, the connective tissue anchors the cardiac muscle cells and is the major component of, and anchor for, the valves (Figs 10.3 and 10.4).

Blood vessels

Blood is pumped away from the heart into arteries which branch and distribute blood, under relatively high pressure, to all regions of the body. Arterial blood passes into smaller arteries (arterioles) and then into very small vessels (capillaries) which have very thin walls (one cell thick). Capillaries are described as exchange vessels because molecules, including carbon dioxide and oxygen, move into and out of capillaries across concentration gradients. In addition,

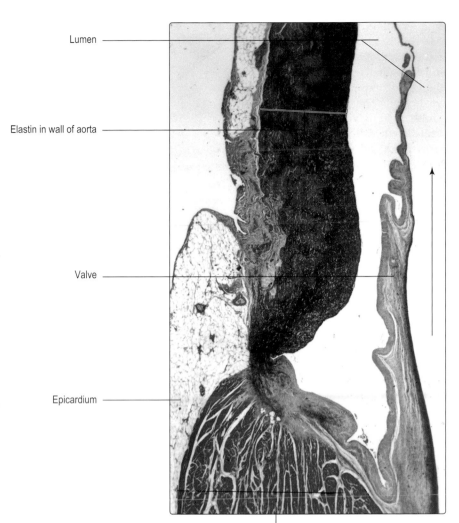

Lumen

Elastin in wall of aorta

Valve

Epicardium

Myocardium of ventricle

Fig. 10.4 **Part of heart wall, a valve and a blood vessel.** An arrow indicates the direction of flow of blood from a ventricle to the blood vessel. The epicardium covering this myocardium appears empty as lipid has been extracted from the adipocytes in the epicardium. (The surface epithelial cells of the epicardium are not resolved at this magnification.) A valve projects into the vessel and is attached to the connective tissue surrounding the myocardium. Elastin, stained brown, in the wall of the blood vessel indicates it is an artery (it is sectioned along its length and only one part of the wall is present). Collagen is stained blue/green. Special stain. Very low magnification.

Clinical notes

Angina This is caused by a slow, but progressive, reduction in the luminal diameter of the coronary arteries that supply blood to the heart and is usually due to the accumulation of fatty material in the walls of these arteries. This process, atheroma formation, may begin as early as 21 years of age as a result of Western-style diets. Angina is manifested by characteristic pain which spreads across the chest wall after exercise. The pain is perceived when insufficient oxygen reaches the cardiac muscle cells and they are unable to sustain the increased rate of contraction needed for the exercise.

Myocardial infarction This is the term used to describe the pathological process of complete or incomplete obstruction of the coronary arteries supplying the heart. The blockage may be due to the deposition of fatty material in the wall of a coronary artery or the presence of a blood clot blocking a coronary artery. Once the blood supply, and therefore oxygen supply, to the cardiac muscle cells is reduced or cut off, the cells die and the patient suffers what is often referred to as a heart attack. If the attack is not fatal the heart may be weakened. The dead muscle cells are not replaced by new muscle cells and connective tissue forms a scar. The normal pattern of heart muscle contraction may be compromised as a result.

nervous system controls the amount of tone (contraction) of the smooth muscle in the walls of arterioles and thus the rate of blood flow to capillaries.

Capillaries

Most capillaries are 4–10 μm in diameter and most are also short in length. They are perfused by blood from arterioles. Networks of branching and connecting (anastomosing) capillaries are present in many regions of the body and are referred to as capillary beds. Capillary walls (Figs 10.9 and 10.10) are formed by a single layer of squamous epithelial cells known as endothelial cells, and their basement membrane (Fig. 10.10). The endothelial cells form the narrow tubes of the capillaries through which blood cells and plasma flow. Around the periphery of some capillaries are pericytes, which have long cytoplasmic processes that wrap around the walls of capillaries. Pericytes contain contractile proteins and thus are able to contract and modify the flow of blood through capillaries. After injury, pericytes are able to differentiate and form new blood vessels and supporting connective tissue.

Although capillaries are very small, they are vital in the functioning of the cardiovascular system as they are the site where exchange of gases, nutrients and waste molecules takes place. They are also important sites where some of the components of blood plasma and white blood cells pass between capillaries and surrounding tissues. Capillaries may be categorised into three groups: continuous, fenestrated or sinusoidal. These groups have significant morphological and functional differences and are present in different locations.

- *Continuous capillaries.* These are located in brain, spinal cord, peripheral nervous tissue, muscle and connective tissues (Fig. 10.9). The endothelial cells lining these capillaries are tightly joined together. Gases diffuse through the endothelial cells and pinocytosis and exocytosis occur in many regions, passing fluid and molecules through the cells.
- *Fenestrated capillaries.* The endothelial cells in these capillaries are tightly joined together but they exhibit tiny pores. These pores are closed by diaphragms formed of cell membranes. This type of capillary is present in endocrine glands and the gastrointestinal tract and allows some

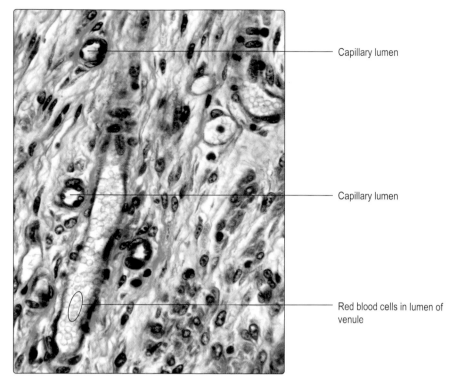

Fig. 10.9 **Capillaries and venules.** Erythrocytes appear as ghostly circles and can be used to estimate the size of the vessels. Connective tissue (green) surrounds the vessels. Special stain. High magnification.

Labels: Capillary lumen; Capillary lumen; Red blood cells in lumen of venule

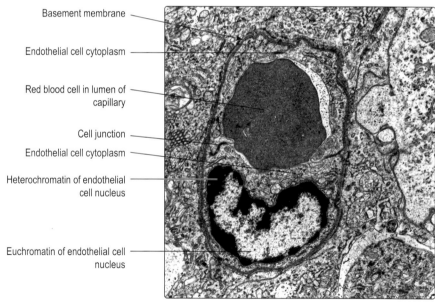

Fig. 10.10 **Electron micrograph of a capillary.** One endothelial cell was sectioned through its nucleus: it displays hetero- and euchromatin. Its cytoplasm is attached to another endothelial cell by a specialised cell junction. The cytoplasm of the attached endothelial cell, not sectioned through its nucleus, extends around the lumen. Low magnification.

Labels: Basement membrane; Endothelial cell cytoplasm; Red blood cell in lumen of capillary; Cell junction; Endothelial cell cytoplasm; Heterochromatin of endothelial cell nucleus; Euchromatin of endothelial cell nucleus

large molecules, e.g. hormones, to pass readily across the capillary walls.
- *Sinusoidal capillaries.* Sinusoidal capillaries differ from other capillaries in that the endothelial cells do not form a continuous layer of tightly attached cells; their basement membrane is also discontinuous. They have fenestrae (openings) in the cytoplasm of endothelial cells and these do not have diaphragms across them. Sinusoids are generally wider in diameter than capillaries and their shape contours around adjacent parenchymal cells. In the walls of some sinusoids, e.g. in the spleen and liver, fixed macrophages are

present. The structure of the walls of sinusoids, in comparison with the walls of other capillaries, facilitates greater opportunities for exchange activities, particularly those involving cells of the immune system.

Veins

Veins are low-pressure blood vessels compared with arteries, and they return blood to the heart. In general, compared with arteries, there is much less smooth muscle and elastin and more collagen in the walls of veins, which accords with the lower pressure within them. Furthermore, the ratio of luminal diameter to wall thickness is greater in veins than in arteries if the comparison is made between vessels adjacent to each other in the body (Fig. 10.11).

Veins may be grouped into three categories according to their size: small, medium and large. The smallest veins, venules, drain capillaries. In medium-sized veins valves are present that prevent the back flow of blood. Valves are flap-like structures which have an endothelial covering and a fibrous core of connective tissue. The flaps project towards the heart; thus, if blood flow to the heart stops, the blood cannot pass backwards because the valve flaps are forced together and close the lumen. Valves are particularly important where there is a need to counteract the force of gravity such as in the limbs. Interestingly, the superficial veins in the lower limbs in humans have a well-developed component of smooth muscle in their walls which, by maintaining muscle tone, is thought to assist in preventing excess distension of the veins due to gravitational forces. The largest veins, close to the heart, do not have valves aiding unidirectional flow. Venous return from large veins below the heart is aided by pressure changes that occur in the thorax during inspiration and gravity aids venous return from the vessels above the heart.

Lymphatic vessels

The lymphatic vessels are an important component of the circulatory system returning some excess extracellular fluid and white blood cells to veins. The smallest lymphatic vessels are lymphatic capillaries. These begin as very small blind-ended tubes formed by endothelial cells. The extracellular (tissue) fluid which drains into lymphatic capillaries is known as lymph. Lymph capillaries resemble blood capillaries but they are characterised by the presence of non-return valves. The pressure in lymphatic vessels is very low and the valves help prevent back flow of lymph. Lymph is carried in lymph vessels to and from lymph nodes (Chapter 8). As lymph passes through lymph nodes immune responses to foreign molecules occur and immune cells such as lymphocytes may be added to the draining lymph (Chapter 8). Lymph draining particular organs and regions of the body passes through specific lymph nodes before draining into wider lymph vessels (lymph ducts). Eventually, the lymph ducts join veins in the neck region and thus lymph is returned to the cardiovascular system.

Fig. 10.11 **Artery and vein.** The wall of this artery contains numerous smooth muscle cells which have been fixed in the contracted state (Chapter 5) and the nuclei of the endothelial cells appear as dark dots projecting into the lumen. Low magnification.

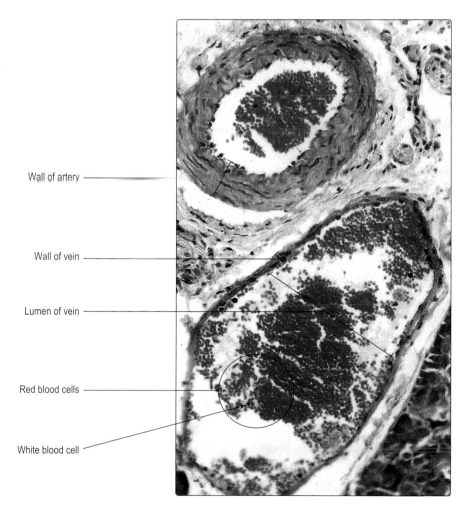

Wall of artery

Wall of vein

Lumen of vein

Red blood cells

White blood cell

Clinical notes

Varicose veins The non-return valves in the superficial veins of the legs may become incompetent, particularly after excess pressure has been sustained such as in pregnancy, or in persons 'on their feet a lot'. When this happens the valves and veins may become dilated and their position becomes apparent as swellings under the skin. These veins may be removed surgically, after which blood finds alternative drainage routes to deeper veins.

Deep vein thrombosis Deep veins accompany the deeply placed arteries in the limbs. These veins are of relatively small calibre and normally venous return is aided by valves. Maintaining tone in the smooth muscle in the walls of these veins helps prevent the veins from distending. In addition, contraction of skeletal muscles in the limb compresses these veins and helps propel the blood towards the heart (as long as the valves are effective). During lengthy periods of inactivity, sufficient venous blood may not be propelled away from the lower limb veins. The blood may become stagnant and clot (i.e. form a thrombus), blocking the deep veins. This causes the limb to swell and become red and painful. The particular danger is that the clot or part of it may detach and pass, via the heart, to the lung, where it may lodge in small blood vessels. This is termed a pulmonary embolism and it can be fatal.

Oedema This is the accumulation of tissue fluid in body tissues which would normally have re-entered venules and lymphatic vessels. It causes swelling of the affected region. It may be part of a local inflammatory reaction or if, for example, it is present in both lower limbs it may be due to increased venous pressure as a result of weak contractions of the right chambers of the heart (right heart failure).

Summary

The circulatory system
- Consists of the heart and the vessels which carry blood or lymph.

The heart
- The heart has paired atria and paired ventricles separated by valves which prevent back flow of blood.
- It has a connective tissue skeleton.
- It is supplied by autonomic nerves which modify the rate at which it beats.
- The myocardium, the middle (thickest) layer, is formed mostly by cardiac muscle cells. Specialised cells (e.g. Purkinje cells) are involved in organising muscle contraction.
- The endocardium, the inner layer, is lined by endothelial cells.
- The epicardium, the outer layer, supports blood vessels supplying the heart, may accumulate fat and is part of the pericardium.

Blood vessels
- These vary in structure and function.
- Arteries (and arterioles) carry blood at relatively high pressure from the heart to capillaries.
- Veins (and venules) carry blood at low pressure from capillaries to the heart. Some veins and venules have valves which aid return of blood to the heart.
- Capillaries have only endothelial cells in their walls and gases, molecules, white blood cells and fluid move across their walls.
- Larger blood vessels have three layers in their walls:
  - tunica intima, the inner layer comprising endothelium and connective tissue
  - tunica media, the middle layer comprising varying amounts of elastin, smooth muscle and collagen
  - tunica adventitia, the outer layer of connective tissue binding vessels to adjacent structures.
- Contraction of smooth muscle in vessel walls is controlled (largely) by sympathetic nerves.

Extracellular (tissue) fluid
- This is formed from plasma.
- Some returns to venules and some to lymphatic capillaries which eventually drain into veins.

Chapter 11
The respiratory system

The function of the respiratory system is to transport gases between the atmosphere and sites in the lungs where gaseous exchange between air and blood occurs. Oxygen diffuses into blood in capillaries in the lungs and carbon dioxide is released from the blood. The respiratory system consists of a series of air-filled passages connecting the nose and mouth to the two lungs in the thorax (Fig. 11.1). Two categories of passages are described, the upper and the lower respiratory tracts. The structure of the walls of the passages of the upper respiratory tract ensures that they do not collapse during breathing. The structure of the walls of the lower respiratory tract ensures that efficient gaseous exchange occurs across a barrier which is 0.1–1.5 µm thick. It is also essential that the passages in the lower respiratory tract do not collapse during respiration.

Whilst the respiratory passages conduct gases through the respiratory system, there are other related structures that help propel the gases along the passages. Each lung is enclosed by a pleural sac formed by a serosal membrane (Fig. 11.1). The visceral layer of the pleura is firmly attached to the surface of each lung and the parietal layer to the inner surface of the chest wall. The pleural cavity (the space enclosed by the pleura) contains fluid secreted by the serosal cells and the lungs are thus able to move during respiration in a relatively friction-free environment. The pleural cavity has an important role in breathing as the pressure in the cavity is less than atmospheric pressure. As the thoracic boundaries (the ribs, intercostal muscles and diaphragm) move during breathing the pleural membranes and lungs move with them. Inspiration increases intrathoracic volume (and the negative pressure in the pleural cavities) and draws air into the lungs. Expiration occurs as the thoracic boundaries decrease intrathoracic volume and stretched elastin fibres in the lung (see below) recoil.

Upper respiratory tract

The upper respiratory tract comprises passages and tubes of decreasing diameter which connect the nose and mouth to the lower respiratory tract in the lungs. From the exterior inwards, the upper respiratory tract comprises the nasal cavity, nasopharynx, larynx, trachea, bronchi and some bronchioles. These passages are also known collectively as the conducting portion of the respiratory tract as they conduct air to the sites of gaseous exchange in the lungs.

During inspiration the upper respiratory passages are under increasing negative pressure as the intrathoracic volume increases. Air will be drawn into the lungs only if the walls of these passages do not collapse. The larger passages have bone or cartilage in their walls which make them relatively rigid and ensure that they remain patent during inspiration. The smallest passages within the lungs, the bronchioles, do not have bone or cartilage in their walls. Bronchioles are held open during inspiration as elastin connective tissue fibres attached to the outer surface of their walls are stretched as a result of the thoracic volume increasing during inspiration.

Most of the upper respiratory tract is lined by a mucosa which consists of a respiratory epithelium and a lamina propria which supports numerous blood vessels. In some regions submucosal connective tissue and aggregations of lymphoid cells are also present. The respiratory epithelium is described as pseudostratified with ciliated columnar epithelial cells and goblet cells (Fig. 11.2). The goblet cells secrete mucus onto the surface of the epithelium and this traps particulate matter which may be harmful. Importantly, the beating motion of cilia of columnar epithelial

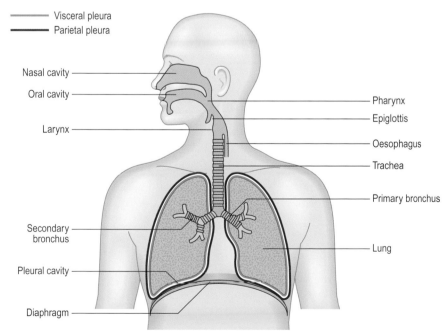

Visceral pleura
Parietal pleura

Nasal cavity
Oral cavity
Larynx
Secondary bronchus
Pleural cavity
Diaphragm

Pharynx
Epiglottis
Oesophagus
Trachea
Primary bronchus
Lung

Fig. 11.1 **The components of the respiratory system including the arrangement of the pleural coverings of the lungs.**

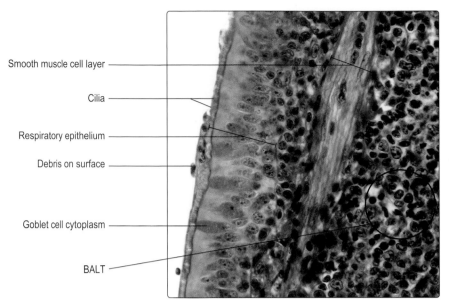

Smooth muscle cell layer

Cilia

Respiratory epithelium

Debris on surface

Goblet cell cytoplasm

BALT

Fig. 11.2 **Bronchus (part of wall).** The mucus in the cytoplasm of goblet cells in the respiratory epithelium is stained pink. BALT, bronchus-associated lymphoid tissue. Special stain. High magnification.

cells moves the mucus so that it is swallowed or discharged from the nose or the mouth. In addition, moisture on the surface of the respiratory epithelium, provided by mucus, humidifies inspired air. This prevents dehydration of the cells lining the lower respiratory tract where gases have to enter an aqueous phase to allow exchange between air and blood. The respiratory epithelium also contains stem cells which can replace damaged goblet and ciliated epithelial cells and replace themselves. Neuroendocrine cells are also present which secrete molecules (paracrine hormones) that regulate the local environment.

Nasal cavities and sinuses

The openings of the nostrils are guarded by short hairs projecting from skin which extends a short distance into the nasal cavity. The hairs are efficient at trapping particles in inspired air. The nasal cavity is separated into left and right sides by a septum, and respiratory epithelium lines most of the cavities. The mucosa lining the cavities is highly vascular and the vessels are vulnerable, hence the risk of epistaxis (nose bleeds). The proximity of blood in vessels to the mucosal surface, particularly in the nasal passages, ensures air is warmed as it travels along the tract. Indeed, air entering the nose at 4°C reaches temperatures not much below blood temperature before arrival at the lower respiratory tract.

Specialised epithelial cells involved in detecting smells, olfactory epithelial cells, lie in the uppermost parts of the nasal cavity. Thus, sniffing odours into the upper part of the nasal cavity is the most efficient way of detecting smells.

Lying adjacent to the nasal cavity are paranasal sinuses. They are four paired structures (the maxillary, frontal, sphenoid and ethmoid sinuses) which open into the nasal cavity. These sinuses are air-filled spaces in skull bones which are lined by respiratory epithelium. The function of the sinuses is unclear, though it may be related to insulating the brain from the effects of inspiring cold air. Other suggested functions include giving resonance to the voice, lightening the weight of the skull and adding to the ability of the upper respiratory tract to 'air condition' (warm and moisten) inhaled air.

In the nasal cavities and the sinuses the mucosa and associated blood vessels are firmly attached to underlying bone or cartilage, and the rigidity conferred by such attachments means that inspiration does not collapse the air passages in these regions.

Nasopharynx

The nasopharynx and the oropharynx are contiguous parts of the pharynx (a large passage shared by the respiratory and the digestive systems). The nasopharynx, which is traversed by air, is lined by respiratory epithelium, but the oropharynx, which carries food (and drink and air) from the mouth, is lined by a stratified squamous epithelium which is able to resist the 'wear and tear' caused by the passage of food.

Aggregations of lymphocytes are a prominent feature deep to the epithe-

lium lining the nasopharynx, particularly on its posterior wall where they form the nasopharyngeal tonsils (adenoids). These aggregations form part of a ring of lymphoid cells (Waldeyer's ring) around the pharynx. Inhaled and ingested antigenic material (e.g. bacteria and viruses) may be trapped in this region and immune responses mounted, thus protecting the respiratory and gastrointestinal tracts from infection.

Larynx

Inspired air passes from the nasopharynx into the larynx and then into the trachea. The larynx has walls containing hyaline cartilage which maintain the patency of the airway, and most of the lumen of the larynx is lined by respiratory epithelium. However, there are flaps (the vocal folds) extending from the walls of the larynx into the lumen which are covered by a stratified squamous epithelium. Vocal cords vibrate and produce sounds and the stratified squamous epithelium resists the wear and tear resulting from the vibrations.

During swallowing, the entry to the larynx from the pharynx is closed temporarily by a large flap-like structure, the epiglottis. This arrangement prevents ingested food and liquid entering the trachea and producing coughing and choking. The stratified squamous epithelium covering the anterior surface of the epiglottis is continuous with the dorsal surface of the tongue and, as it is in contact with food during swallowing is subject to abrasion. In contrast, the posterior surface of the epiglottis is exposed only to air and is covered by respiratory epithelium. The flexibility and recoil movements of the epiglottis during swallowing are aided by its core of elastic cartilage (see Fig. 9.1).

Trachea

The trachea is a tube attached to the larynx in the neck and it extends about 10 cm into the thorax. It is 2–3 cm in diameter and is kept patent by 15 to 20 incomplete 'C'-shaped rings of hyaline cartilage in its wall (Fig. 11.3). Each ring of cartilage is completed on the posterior wall of the trachea by smooth muscle and connective tissue containing elastin fibres. The trachea is lined by respiratory epithelium (Fig. 11.3) and there are serous and mucous glands (Fig. 11.4) in submucosal connective tissue. Secretions from the submucosal glands and goblet cells in the epithelium are propelled by ciliary

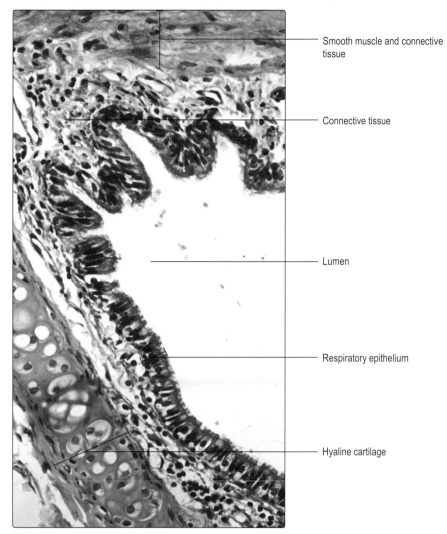

Fig. 11.3 **Trachea (part of wall).** Medium magnification.

- Smooth muscle and connective tissue
- Connective tissue
- Lumen
- Respiratory epithelium
- Hyaline cartilage

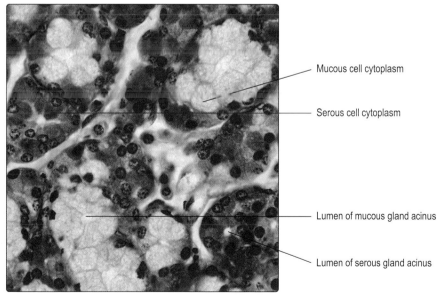

Fig. 11.4 **Serous and mucous glands.** Special stain. High magnification.

- Mucous cell cytoplasm
- Serous cell cytoplasm
- Lumen of mucous gland acinus
- Lumen of serous gland acinus

activity toward the pharynx and are usually swallowed.

Bronchi

The trachea bifurcates into two main (primary) bronchi (Fig. 11.1). These enter the lungs and divide into lobar (secondary) bronchi. Each of these subdivides about 10 times into segmental (tertiary) bronchi which supply specific areas of lung known as bronchopulmonary segments. Each of these segments of lung has its own branch of a pulmonary artery as well as a single tertiary bronchus, and each has clinical significance. For example, knowledge of the architecture of bronchopulmonary segments is vital in bronchoscopy. In addition, a disease may be confined to one segment of lung and surgical resection may be used to remove the diseased segment. Further branching of bronchi in segments reduces their diameter to 5 mm and, at this dimension, branching continues but the passages are then known as bronchioles.

All bronchi contain hyaline cartilage in their walls which maintains their patency. Primary bronchi have, like the trachea, incomplete rings of cartilage in their walls. Intrapulmonary branches of bronchi have irregularly placed plates of cartilage in their walls (Fig. 11.5). Large bronchi are lined by respiratory epithelium (Fig. 11.5), but as they become smaller in diameter gradual changes occur in the epithelium (see below). The submucosal layer of bronchi contains serous and mucous glands which secrete onto the epithelial surface (Fig. 11.6). Secretions on the epithelial surface are moved up the 'mucus escalator' to the pharynx by ciliary activity of the columnar epithelial cells. Smooth muscle (Figs 11.2 and 11.6) is also present in the walls of bronchi and the muscle cells are arranged spirally along the length of the walls. Parasympathetic stimulation of this smooth muscle causes contraction which reduces the diameter of the lumen. Conversely, sympathetic nerve stimulation relaxes the muscle and increases the diameter of the airway. The strength of muscle contraction is not great enough to collapse the bronchi because of the relatively rigid cartilage lying outside the muscle layer. Aggregations of lymphocytes are a common feature in the walls of bronchi (Figs 11.2 and 11.5) and are described as 'bronchus-associated lymphoid tissue' (BALT). In these regions, interactions between macrophages and lymphocytes take place which are important in immune defence of the lungs.

Bronchioles

Bronchioles, passages of less than 5 mm in diameter, do not have cartilage in their walls but have smooth muscle (Fig. 11.7). The patency of bronchioles during inspiration is assisted not by cartilage in their walls but by elastin fibres in surrounding connective tissue attached to the bronchioles which are stretched as

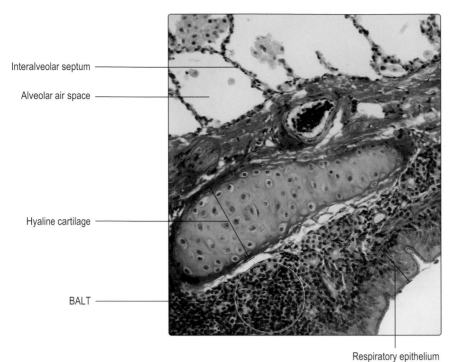

Interalveolar septum

Alveolar air space

Hyaline cartilage

BALT

Respiratory epithelium

Fig. 11.5 **Bronchus (part of wall) and alveoli.** Medium magnification.

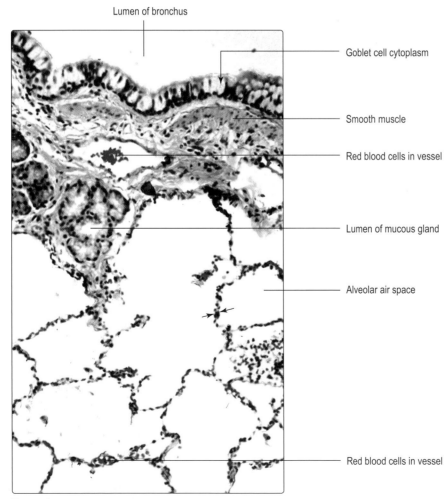

Lumen of bronchus

Goblet cell cytoplasm

Smooth muscle

Red blood cells in vessel

Lumen of mucous gland

Alveolar air space

Red blood cells in vessel

Fig. 11.6 **Bronchus (part of wall) and lung alveoli.** Arrows show the width of an interalveolar septum. Erythrocytes appear as bright red dots; some are visible in the septa. Connective tissue is blue/green. Special stain. Low magnification.

the thoracic volume is increased during inspiration and air is drawn into the respiratory tract.

Smooth muscle cells spiral around bronchioles deep to the epithelium and their contraction affects the diameter of these airways. The state of contraction of this smooth muscle is the major factor affecting the volume of air reaching the lower, respiratory portion of the tract. Parasympathetic nerve impulses cause these muscle cells to contract and this reduces the diameter of the bronchioles and thus restricts air flow. Conversely, sympathetic nerve impulses relax the muscle cells and this aids air flow. Indeed, malfunction of this smooth muscle in asthma so that airways constrict, significantly reduces the volume of air entering the lungs and results in the distressing and serious effects of the disease.

As the conducting tubes of the respiratory system reduce in calibre, the type of lining epithelium gradually changes. Instead of the typical respiratory epithelium (pseudostratified, ciliated columnar, with goblet cells) as in the larger bronchi (Figs 11.2, 11.5 and 11.6), they become lined by a simple epithelium. Most bronchioles are lined by a simple epithelium consisting of ciliated columnar cells and a few goblet cells. Smaller divisions of bronchioles are lined by ciliated low columnar or cuboidal cells (Fig. 11.7); goblet cells are not present in the smaller bronchioles. In terminal bronchioles the epithelium may become flattened taking on a squamous appearance (Fig. 11.8). There are also specialised cells (Clara cells) in the epithelium lining the smallest bronchioles which may serve a protective function. (Clara cells are prominent in some non-human species.)

There are no submucous glands in bronchioles and very few goblet cells. If such glands and goblet cells were present, it could lead to too much fluid in the bronchioles which may drain into and 'drown' the gaseous exchange region of the lower respiratory tract.

Lower respiratory tract

The most distal, lower part of the respiratory tract is also described as the respiratory portion of the tract as it is here that gaseous exchange between air and blood occurs. The walls of the passages are at their thinnest and this facilitates the exchange of gases. Terminal bronchioles continue as respiratory bronchioles. In some parts of respiratory bronchioles the epithelium is simple cuboidal, but in other parts squamous epithelial cells are present and gaseous exchange occurs across the cells in these regions.

Respiratory bronchioles open into alveolar ducts, which in turn lead to several alveoli (Fig. 11.8). Some alveoli are adjacent to each other and share their walls. These walls are known as interalveolar septa (Figs 11.5–11.8). There are several hundred million alveoli per lung offering an enormous surface area where gaseous exchange occurs.

The epithelium lining alveoli lies very close to a capillary network and it is across this air–blood barrier that gases, in the aqueous phase, diffuse. The barrier between air and blood is very thin (Figs 11.6 and 11.7) and consists of (Fig. 11.9):

■ an alveolar epithelium and its basement membrane
■ connective tissue (sparse)
■ a capillary endothelium and its basement membrane.

The alveolar epithelium comprises type I and type II pneumocytes. Type I pneumocytes make up the majority of the surface of alveoli and their cytoplasm forms a very thin layer closely applied to the basement membrane: this aids the diffusion of gases. Type II pneumocytes are roughly spherical cells which synthesise and secrete a surfactant (a lipid material with detergent-like qualities) which reduces surface tension in the alveoli. During inspiration this low surface tension makes it easier to draw air into the alveoli and helps to prevent the alveoli from collapsing.

The connective tissue around alveoli is sparse (Figs 11.6 and 11.7) and consists mainly of elastin fibres, although a little collagen is present. The elastin fibres are stretched on inspiration and this helps to draw air into the alveoli. Importantly, recoil of the elastin during expiration helps to expel air from the alveoli. In some regions there is no connective tissue and the basement membranes of an alveolar epithelium and the adjacent capillary endothelium are fused, thus reducing the distance gases have to travel between air and blood (Fig. 11.9).

Throughout the lungs a variety of immune cells are present. These include cells which phagocytose particulate matter, including bacteria, and others which mount immune responses to foreign molecules. Lying on the alveoli, on the air side or apparently lying free within the air space, are alveolar macrophages. These cells are also present within interalveolar septa. Some macrophages may migrate onto the surface of the epithelium and others may remain in the lungs throughout life. Macrophages are particularly apparent if they have ingested inert particles such as carbon and this can give lungs a black appearance at post-mortem examination.

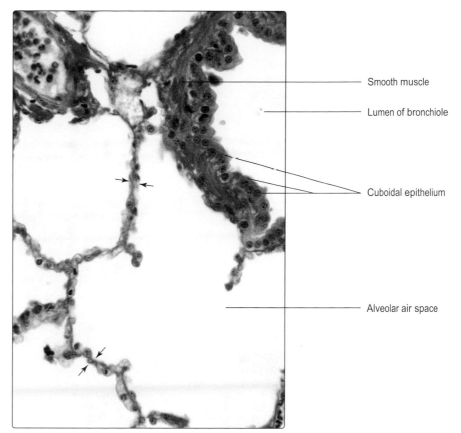

Fig. 11.7 **Bronchiole (part of wall) and lung alveoli.** Arrows show the width of two interalveolar septa. Connective tissue is red. Special stain. High magnification.

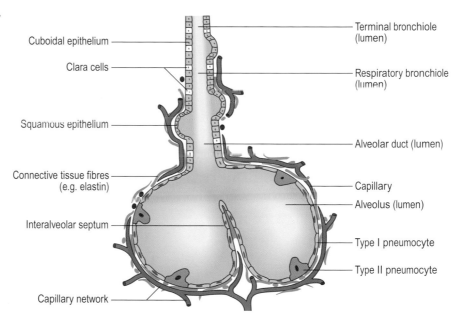

Fig. 11.8 **The microscopic structure of the terminal components of the airway.**

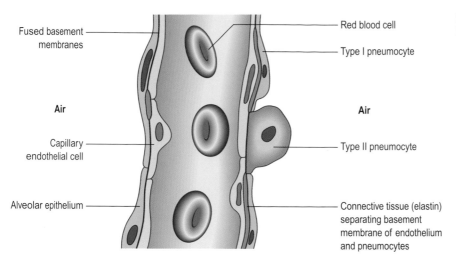

Fused basement membranes

Red blood cell

Type I pneumocyte

Air

Air

Capillary endothelial cell

Type II pneumocyte

Alveolar epithelium

Connective tissue (elastin) separating basement membrane of endothelium and pneumocytes

Fig. 11.9 **The microscopic structure of the blood–air barrier.**

Clinical notes

Infantile respiratory distress syndrome Prior to 28 weeks of development in utero, type II pneumocytes are unable to synthesise surfactant and, as a consequence, alveoli do not fill with air on inspiration; as a result, premature infants may not survive. In addition, the alveolar wall before about 26 weeks of development is insufficiently thin to enable gaseous exchange.

Smoking Goblet cells increase in number and ciliated cells decrease in number in smokers. One consequence is mucus is not cleared readily from the respiratory passages. Coughing may help clear the passages and prevent mucus from reaching the alveoli and decreasing the efficiency of gaseous exchange. Smoking is associated with an increased risk of heart disease and lung cancer.

Asthma In this condition the airways are abnormally constricted by contraction of the smooth muscle, particularly in the bronchioles. It is often a consequence of immune (allergic) reactions. In asthmatics the airways are inflamed and produce excessive amounts of mucus. Attacks are usually acute episodes of wheezing, coughing and difficulty in breathing. These episodes may be effectively treated with inhalers containing drugs which dilate the airways, and steroid-based drugs which reduce the inflammation.

Cystic fibrosis This is an inherited condition in which excessive amounts of viscous mucus are produced. It is often thought of as a purely respiratory disorder but it is a disorder of exocrine glands. The excess secretions of the exocrine glands cause obstruction in the lungs and a range of other organs such as the pancreas, liver and intestines. The disease pursues a chronic course and sufferers rarely live beyond their third decade.

Summary

- The respiratory system consists of the lungs and a series of passages carrying air to them:
  - the upper respiratory tract passages transport air to and from the lower respiratory tract, where exchange of gases (oxygen and carbon dioxide) between blood and air occurs.
- The chest wall, diaphragm and pleural membranes around the lungs are involved in moving air in and out of the lungs (during inspiration and expiration).
- The walls of the trachea and bronchi contain hyaline cartilage which provides rigidity and prevents the passages collapsing during inspiration:
  - all these passage are lined by the typical respiratory epithelium.
- The walls of bronchioles do not contain cartilage and they are kept open during inspiration as elastin fibres attached to their walls are stretched:
  - the respiratory epithelium is gradually replaced in bronchioles by a simple columnar or cuboidal (non-ciliated) epithelium.
- Smooth muscle is present in the walls of bronchi and bronchioles and is controlled by autonomic nerves.
- The walls of the lower respiratory tract are extremely thin and gaseous exchange occurs mostly in alveoli.
- The blood–air barrier in alveoli comprises:
  - endothelial cells and their basement membrane, sparse elastin fibres, alveolar epithelial cells and their basement membrane
  - alveolar epithelium is formed mostly by very flattened cells (type I pneumocytes), and some type II pneumocytes which are rounded and secrete surfactant.
- Aggregations of immune cells are present in the walls of the respiratory tract and macrophages are present in alveolar walls and on the surface of the alveolar epithelium.

Chapter 12
The digestive system

The digestive system consists of the alimentary canal, which is a tube connecting the mouth and anus, and associated structures that facilitate digestion of ingested food and drink (Fig. 12.1). The alimentary canal comprises the mouth, oesophagus and gastrointestinal tract. The gastrointestinal tract comprises the stomach, duodenum, jejunum, ileum, colon, appendix, rectum and the upper part of the anal canal. The associated structures are the teeth, tongue, salivary glands, liver and pancreas. At the mouth, lips intervene between skin and the mouth and they are covered by a stratified squamous epithelium which is not keratinised. At the anus the stratified, keratinised squamous epithelium of skin extends a short distance into the anal canal. The upper part of the anal canal is lined by a stratified, squamous epithelium which is not keratinised.

The digestive system has two primary functions. It breaks down food and drink into small molecules such as glucose, amino acids, fatty acids and triglycerides, a process which involves enzymic activity and is known as digestion. The second primary function of the digestive system ensures the small molecules produced by digestion in the lumen of the alimentary canal enter the body 'proper' by being absorbed across the epithelium lining the alimentary canal and into the blood or lymphatic vessels. In addition, the digestive system absorbs water, minerals, vitamins and ions from the material in the lumen of the gastrointestinal tract. The terminal part of the tract functions as a store for components of food that have not been digested. The stored, undigested food and waste products of the body, e.g. from the breakdown of red blood cells, are emptied from the alimentary canal at defecation.

The structure of the alimentary canal is related to its functions and different aspects of function occur at different locations along the canal. The gastrointestinal tract itself is several metres in length in humans, which is a reflection of the space required to accomplish all aspects of its function and is related to the transit times required for these functions.

General structure of the alimentary canal

All the alimentary canal is lined by a mucosa (Chapter 3), which consists of an epithelium, connective tissue lamina propria and, in many regions, a layer of smooth muscle forming the muscularis mucosae (Fig. 12.2). The epithelium of the mucosa reflects the primary function(s) occurring in that region. However, in all regions the mucosa is important in forming a barrier between substances ingested, including microorganisms, and the internal environment of the body. In regions where the muscularis mucosae is present, contraction of this muscle moves and folds the mucosa, aiding contact between the contents of the lumen and the surface epithelial cells.

A submucosal layer of connective tissue, which supports nerves and blood and lymph vessels, attaches the mucosa in most parts of the alimentary canal to outer layers of muscle (the muscularis externa) (Fig. 12.2). In most regions of the alimentary canal two layers of muscle are present in the muscularis externa. In the outer, longitudinal layer the long axis of each muscle cell lies roughly parallel to the length of the lumen. In the inner, circular layer the long axes of the muscle cells lie around

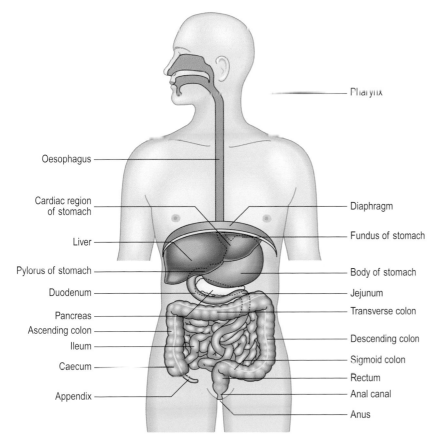

Fig. 12.1 **Components of the digestive system.**

Labels:
- Pharynx
- Oesophagus
- Cardiac region of stomach
- Liver
- Pylorus of stomach
- Duodenum
- Pancreas
- Ascending colon
- Ileum
- Caecum
- Appendix
- Diaphragm
- Fundus of stomach
- Body of stomach
- Jejunum
- Transverse colon
- Descending colon
- Sigmoid colon
- Rectum
- Anal canal
- Anus

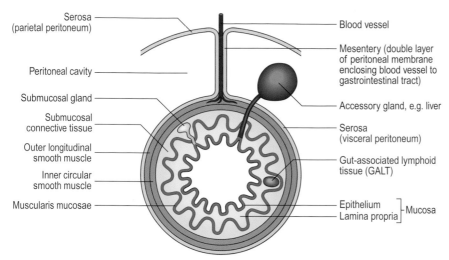

Fig. 12. 2 **Generalised transverse section through the gastrointestinal tract.** The outer and inner smooth muscle layers form the muscularis externa.

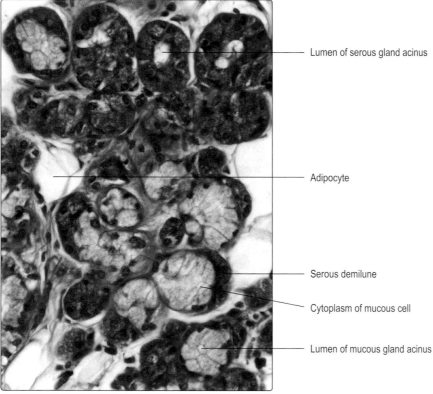

Fig. 12.3 **Submandibular gland, serous and mucous glands.** The carbohydrate content in the cytoplasm of mucous gland cells is palely stained and the protein content of serous cells is darkly stained. Empty spaces are where lipid in adipocytes has been extracted. Medium magnification.

the lumen. Contractions of the muscularis externa cause peristalsis, which provides the motive force transporting the luminal contents of the canal towards the anus. In the submucosal layer and the muscularis externa, parasympathetic neuronal cell bodies are present and some are involved in co-ordinating muscle activity.

In some regions of the alimentary canal the muscularis externa is attached to adjacent structures by connective tissue known as the adventitia. However, in most regions of the canal in the abdomi-nal cavity, the muscularis externa is covered by a serosal membrane (Chapter 3) which is the inner (visceral) layer of the peritoneum. The visceral peritoneal membrane is continuous with the parietal peritoneal membrane, which is attached to the abdominal walls (and part of the liver). Squamous epithelial cells on the surface of the peritoneal membranes secrete small amounts of fluid into the peritoneal cavity. The surface of perito-neal membranes is kept moist by these secretions, which provide lubrication to ensure that, as gut tubes move against each other, potentially damaging friction does not occur. In addition, the peritoneal membranes enclose the vessels and nerves supplying the gut tube.

Specialised gut-associated lymphoid tissue (GALT) is present in the walls of the alimentary canal. In some regions, GALT forms large structures, e.g. tonsils; in other regions, only small clusters of lymphoid cells are present (Fig. 12.2). These cells are part of the primary defence mechanisms against pathogens entering the body across the mucosa lining the gut tube.

Mouth

The mouth (oral cavity) contains the tongue and teeth. The epithelium of the mucosa lining the cheeks and tongue is able to resist the wear and tear in-volved in chewing food, and in most regions it is a stratified, squamous (non-keratinised) epithelium. This epithelial surface is moistened by secretions from small serous and mucous glands in the submucosal layer and from salivary glands (Fig. 12.3) which drain their saliva into the oral cavity. Physical break-down of food occurs in the mouth and it is mixed with salivary gland secretions which begin to break down large carbo-hydrate molecules.

Salivary glands

There are three, paired salivary glands, the parotid, submandibular and sub-lingual glands. Each gland is invested by a connective tissue capsule, and connec-tive tissue forms trabeculae which pen-etrate the glands and provide support for the blood vessels and nerves supply-ing the glands and for the ducts drain-ing them. Each gland has secretory cells arranged as compound, tubuloacinar, exocrine glands (Chapter 3). The secre-tory acini drain into small ducts (lined by a simple cuboidal epithelium) which join together in a branching system; the larger ducts are lined by columnar epi-thelial cells, which may be stratified. The ducts drain the saliva into the oral cavity.

Two types of secretory cell, serous and mucous cells, are present in salivary gland acini (Fig. 12.3) and, respectively, they produce a watery secretion contain-ing proteins which function as enzymes and a viscous mucus in which large carbohydrate complexes are major com-ponents. In addition, myoepithelial cells wrap around the acini and their contrac-tions help to expel the secretions. The secretions assist the process of digestion by moistening and lubricating the food, and by providing enzymes. The main enzyme is amylase, which breaks down large carbohydrate molecules. Saliva is also responsible for lubricating and cleansing the oral cavity. It contains bactericidal substances such as lysozyme secreted by serous cells and may contain immunoglobulin A secreted by plasma cells.

Parotid glands

The parotid glands are the largest of the salivary glands. Each parotid gland is located close to an ear, and each duct drains into the oral cavity near the ipsilateral second upper molar tooth. Serous cells line the acini and form the majority of the parenchyma of the parotid glands (Fig. 12.4). Adipose cells appear in the parotid glands with age. Many small ducts are distributed throughout the parenchyma of parotid glands and they are lined by epithelial cells which stain readily with eosin (Fig. 12.4).

Submandibular glands

A submandibular gland lies beneath the mandible on each side, wrapped around the muscle which supports the tongue. Each gland drains via a duct that opens on the ipsilateral side of the ridge (the frenulum) on the undersurface of the tongue. Mucous glands are a prominent feature of submandibular glands, but serous cells are also present. The arrangement of the serous and mucous gland cells together in some acini is such that these are described as mucous glands with serous demilunes (Fig. 12.3).

Sublingual glands

The sublingual glands are the smallest of the salivary glands. Mucous gland cells are predominant in sublingual glands and the ducts open directly into the floor of the oral cavity, rather than via a single duct system.

Tongue

The tongue is covered by a stratified, non-keratinised, squamous epithelium which on the undersurface is similar to the epithelium lining the mouth. The upper surface of the tongue is divided by a 'V'-shaped groove into an anterior (two-thirds) and a posterior region developed from different parts of the embryo (see Mitchell B, Sharma R. *Embryology: An Illustrated Colour Text.* Elsevier: 2004). The stratified squamous epithelium on the upper surface is studded by prominent projections. In the posterior region, many of the projections are due to aggregations of lym-

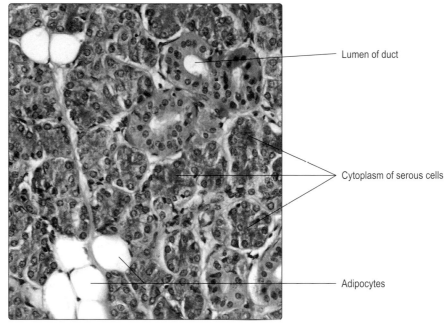

Fig. 12.4 **Parotid gland.** Medium magnification.

phocytes deep to the epithelium. In addition, three distinct types of projection known as papillae are also described, and all assist in macerating food and resisting abrasion:

- *Filiform papillae.* These are numerous on the upper surface and are in parallel rows which converge towards the midline. The surface of these papillae is covered by a keratinised, stratified squamous epithelium.
- *Fungiform papillae.* These are covered by a stratified (non-keratinised) squamous epithelium. Specialised clusters of sensory cells (taste buds) are present in the epithelium covering this type of papilla.
- *Circumvallate papillae.* There are 8 to 12 large, circumvallate papillae visible to the unaided eye just anterior to the 'V'-shaped groove of the tongue. They are also covered by a stratified (non-keratinised) squamous epithelium which contains taste buds.

Deep to the mucosa of the tongue there are numerous, small serous and mucous glands which secrete onto the surface of the epithelium. The major component of the inner part of the tongue is skeletal muscle (see Fig. 5.7). The bundles of muscle cells are arranged in a complex three-dimensional meshwork and coordinated contraction of the muscle cells is important in chewing, swallowing and in sound production.

Pharynx and oesophagus

Swallowed food and drink pass via the pharynx to the oesophagus (gullet). The structure and function of the epithelium lining the component parts of the pharynx are described in Chapter 11. Aggregations of lymphoid cells are a prominent feature of the walls of the pharynx and form tonsils (Fig. 12.5). The lymphoid cells are important components of the immune mechanisms defending the alimentary canal (and the respiratory tract).

The major part of the oesophagus is in the thorax, but a small segment lies in the abdominal cavity and is continuous with the stomach. The structures in the walls of the oesophagus conform to the general plan for the gastrointestinal tract (Fig. 12.2). In the thorax, the connective tissue of the adventitia binds the muscularis externa of the oesophagus to adjacent structures. The muscularis externa consists of an outer, approximately longitudinal layer and an inner circular layer. In the upper part of the muscularis externa, striated voluntary muscle (Fig. 12.6) is present, whereas in the lower region it is replaced by smooth involuntary muscle. In the middle region there is a transition between the two types of muscle. Coordinated contraction of muscle cells in the different regions of the oesophagus ensures that swallowed food and drink normally pass to the stomach. In some regions, the submucosal tissue of the oesophagus contains serous and mucous glands in addition to

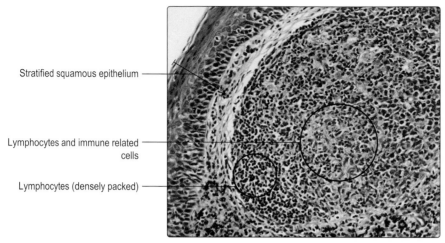

Stratified squamous epithelium

Lymphocytes and immune related cells

Lymphocytes (densely packed)

Fig. 12.5 **Tonsil.** This displays a secondary lymphoid follicle as there are palely stained cells in the centre of a follicle indicating an immune response was occurring. Lymphocytes at the edge of the follicle are densely packed. The epithelium covering the tonsil is typical of the oropharynx. Low magnification.

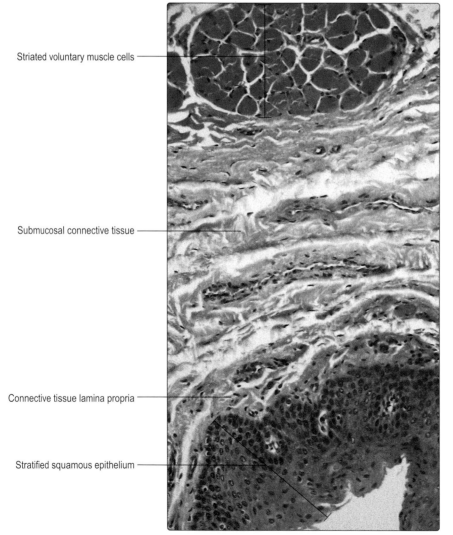

Striated voluntary muscle cells

Submucosal connective tissue

Connective tissue lamina propria

Stratified squamous epithelium

Fig. 12.6 **Oesophagus, upper region.** Striated voluntary muscle cells can be identified by the peripheral position of their nuclei. The distinction between the connective tissue forming the layers of lamina propria and submucosa is not possible at this magnification. Low magnification.

blood vessels, nerves and aggregations of lymphoid cells. The epithelium of the mucosa lining the oesophagus is stratified and squamous (Fig. 12.6) and is able to resist friction from swallowed food and chemical attack by swallowed drinks, e.g. alcohol.

The gastrointestinal tract

Stomach

The stomach is a dilated portion of the gastrointestinal tract. It is described as having four regions: the cardiac region, the fundus, the body and the pylorus (Fig. 12.1). The cardiac region is continuous with the lower end of the oesophagus. The fundus is the part of the stomach lying closest to the diaphragm and is a site, in humans, where gas collects. The body of the stomach is the largest part of the stomach and the pylorus connects the body of the stomach to the duodenum. The stomach produces 2–3 litres/day of gastric secretions (juices) and the main constituents are mucus, water, hydrochloric acid and enzymes able to digest carbohydrates, fats and proteins. The mixture of gastric juices and ingested food and drink is known as chyme. The structure of the stomach conforms to the general plan (Fig. 12.2) with some modifications which relate to its functions.

The stomach is covered by a serosal (peritoneal) membrane. The surface squamous epithelial cells of the peritoneal membrane secrete small amounts of fluid (into the peritoneal cavity) and, as the stomach fills with food and drink, it moves relatively easily against adjacent structures. Within the connective tissue of the peritoneal membrane large accumulations of fat cells may be present. The muscularis externa of the stomach differs from the general plan in that it has three layers: an innermost oblique, a middle circular and an outer longitudinal layer. These muscle layers help prevent overdistension of the stomach and their contractions help mix the chyme and move it towards the small intestine. In the pyloric region of the stomach, at the gastroduodenal junction, the muscularis externa is thickened and functions as a sphincter. The sphincter is controlled by autonomic nerves and hormones which regulate the passage of chyme into the duodenum. In contrast, at the gastro-oesophageal junction, stomach contents normally are not regurgitated into the oesophagus although a distinct muscular sphincter is not apparent.

The interior of the empty stomach is characterised by thick folds which run longitudinally. They are known as rugae and are formed by submucosal and mucosal layers. The rugae unfold as the stomach fills. They also help to channel chyme towards the pylorus and help to maintain a large interface between the contents of the stomach and the surface epithelium.

The gastric mucosa has a simple epithelium which contains a variety of cell types and it is supported by a sparse lamina propria. The underlying muscularis mucosae is atypical in that it has three layers of smooth muscle. It actively moves the mucosa, thus increasing contact between mucosa, gastric juices and ingested substances.

The epithelium of the gastric mucosa dips into the lamina propria and forms channels known as gastric pits (Fig. 12.7). All the epithelial cells on the surface of all regions of the stomach and lining all the gastric pits are columnar and they secrete mucus (Fig. 12.8). This mucus forms a thick protective layer which helps to ensure that the stomach cells are not damaged by gastric secretions. At the base of the pits, gastric glands extend as tubes deep into the lamina propria and reach the muscularis mucosae. The gastric glands secrete various substances which drain into the pits, and from there to the lumen of the stomach. In the cardiac and pyloric regions of the stomach gastric glands are coiled tubules lined by columnar cells which secrete mucus. Their appearance in routine H&E-stained sections resembles the mucous cells lining gastric pits. In the rest of the stomach (body and fundus) the gastric glands are straight tubules and the epithelium lining them contains several types of cell:

- *Zymogenic (chief) cells* (Fig. 12.9). These produce and secrete pepsinogen (and lipase, which digests lipids). Pepsinogen is inactive until it is converted by the acidity of the gastic juices, into pepsin, which breaks proteins down into smaller molecules. The release of gastric enzymes is stimulated by the vagus nerve, which is part of the parasympathetic nervous system.
- *Oxyntic (parietal) cells* (Fig. 12.9). These produce and secrete hydrochloric acid, which helps provide the optimum pH for enzymes secreted by zymogenic cells. The acid also destroys some

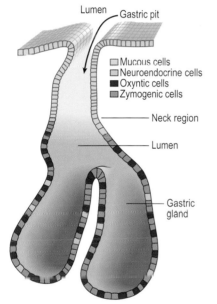

Fig. 12.7 **Epithelial cells lining a gastric pit and gastric glands (typical of the fundus and body region).**

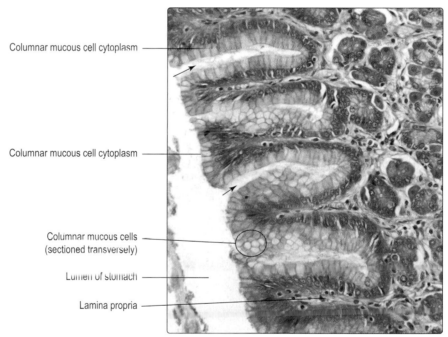

Fig. 12.8 **Stomach, body region showing gastric pits.** Arrows show the entrance to pits. Medium magnification.

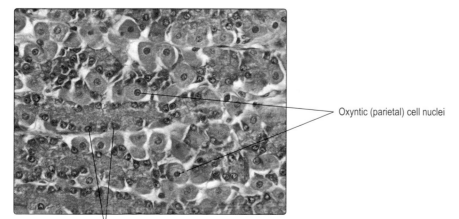

Fig. 12.9 **Stomach, body region showing gastric glands.** The eosinophilic cytoplasm of oxyntic cells distinguishes them from the basophilic cytoplasm of the zymogenic cells. Large numbers of mitochondria in the cytoplasm of oxyntic cells and large amounts of cytoplasmic RNA in zymogenic cells account for the difference in staining. Medium magnification.

ingested microorganisms. Secretion of acid is stimulated by the vagus nerve too. Oxyntic cells also secrete intrinsic factor, which is necessary for the absorption of vitamin B12, which is essential, in turn, for the production of red blood cells. Without intrinsic factor pernicious anaemia develops.

- *Mucous neck cells*. These are columnar cells near to the junction of gastric pits and glands and they secrete mucus.
- *Stem cells*. These are located amongst the mucous neck cells and, although relatively few in number, are able to undergo mitosis and give rise to replacement gastric epithelial cells of all types. Some offspring cells differentiate and migrate into their appropriate location within the epithelium; others remain as stem cells.
- *Neuroendocrine cells*. These secrete a variety of hormones into the local environment and into blood vessels that modify the activity of other cells. For example, in the mucosa of the stomach some cells secrete gastrin, which stimulates contraction of the muscularis externa of the stomach and relaxation of the pyloric sphincter, thus moving stomach contents into the duodenum.

Small intestine

The small intestine has three parts: duodenum, jejunum and ileum. Digestion continues in the small intestine and involves digestive enzymes from secretory cells in the mucosal epithelium and, in the duodenum, in the submucosa. Secretions also enter the lumen of the duodenum from the pancreas and liver and these also aid digestion. The luminal contents, known as chyle, have a transit time along the small intestine of 3–4 hours and digestion is largely completed in that time. Most of the products of digestion, e.g. amino acids and monosaccharides, are absorbed across the epithelium lining the small intestine and pass into blood vessels; fatty acids and triglycerides pass into lacteals (small, blind-ended lymph vessels).

The wall of the small intestine conforms to the generalized structural plan of the gastrointestinal tract (Fig. 12.2) though there are features which characterise each part. The epithelium of the mucosa lining the small intestine contains:

- columnar epithelial cells (Fig. 12.10), which are specialised for absorption of small molecules from the lumen (see below)
- goblet cells, which make and secrete mucus that helps to protect the luminal surface (Fig. 12.10)
- Paneth cells, which make, store and secrete lysozyme (Fig. 12.11)
- neuroendocrine cells, which secrete molecules that affect the function of other cells
- stem cells (Fig. 12.11) (see below)
- lymphocytes, which may be between the epithelial cells (Fig. 12.10).

Clinical note

Stomach ulcer Some stomach ulcers are the result of damage to epithelial cells lining the stomach by specific molecules, e.g. alcohol or aspirin. If epithelial cells are killed by such molecules the damage may be repaired by the normal proliferative activity of stem cells in the epithelium. However, if the damage is extensive and the production of replacement cells inadequate, the damage may extend into the connective tissue lamina propria and bleeding into the gastric lumen may occur.

There are several structural features of the small intestine that facilitate contact between luminal contents and the mucosal epithelium and thus aid digestion and absorption of the molecules produced by enzymic activities:

- *Transverse folds*. These are visible in the duodenum, jejunum and first half of the ileum to the unaided eye. These folds are formed by the mucosa and submucosa and are known as plicae circulares.
- *Villi* (Figs 12.12 and 12.13). These are present throughout the small intestine and are microscopic finger-like structures which project from

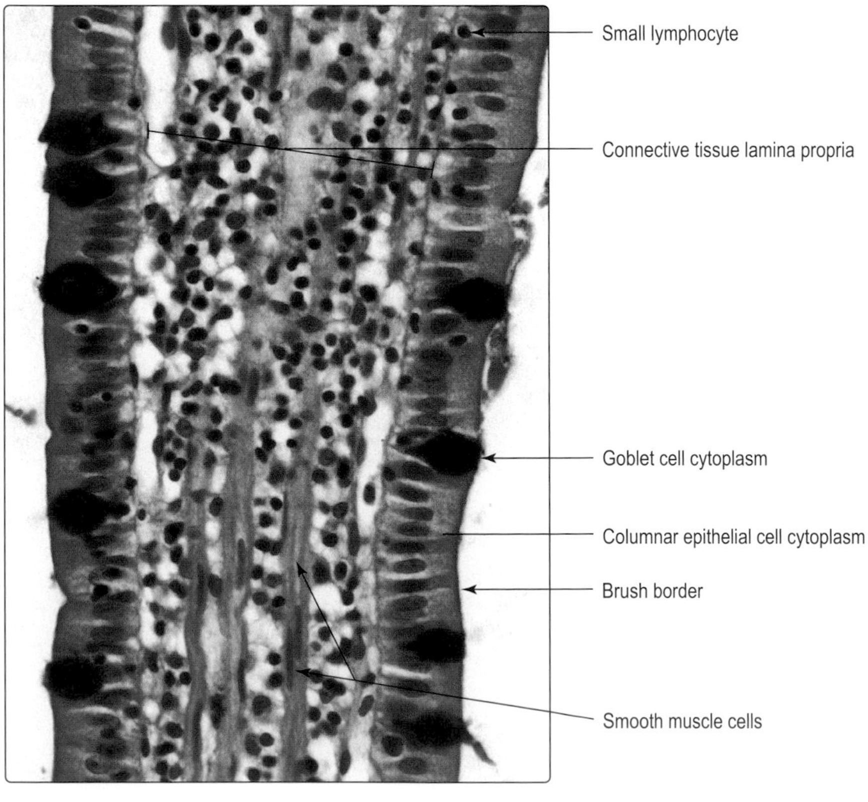

Fig. 12.10 **Small intestine, part of villus sectioned along its length.** The brush border represents the microvilli increasing the surface area of the absorptive, columnar epithelial cells. The mucus in the goblet cells is stained blue. Special stain. High magnification.

Small lymphocyte

Connective tissue lamina propria

Goblet cell cytoplasm

Columnar epithelial cell cytoplasm

Brush border

Smooth muscle cells

Fig. 12.11 **Small intestine, base of intestinal gland.** Cells undergoing mitosis have characteristically condensed chromatin. In the base of intestinal glands stem cells divide and one in the anaphase stage of mitosis (Chapter 2) is displayed. Paneth cells are distinguished by their position at the base of the intestinal glands and their eosinophilic granules. High magnification.

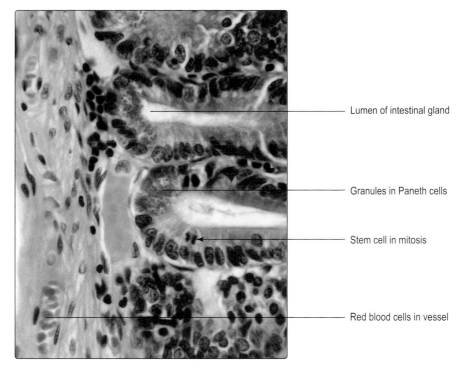

— Lumen of intestinal gland

— Granules in Paneth cells

— Stem cell in mitosis

— Red blood cells in vessel

Fig. 12.12 **Small intestine, intestinal glands and part of a villus sectioned along its length.** Special stain. Low magnification.

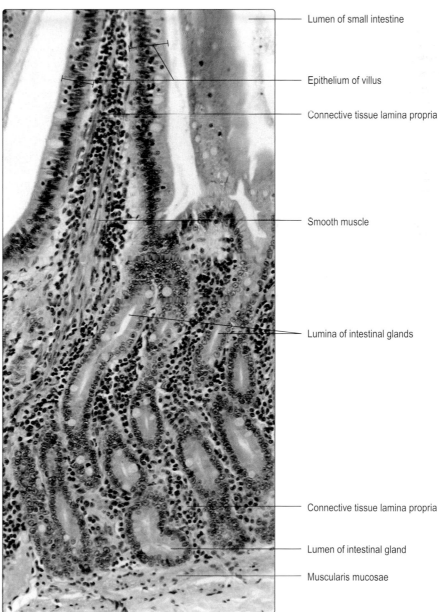

— Lumen of small intestine

— Epithelium of villus

— Connective tissue lamina propria

— Smooth muscle

— Lumina of intestinal glands

— Connective tissue lamina propria

— Lumen of intestinal gland

— Muscularis mucosae

the mucosa into the lumen (Figs 12.12 and 12.13). They are covered by columnar epithelial absorptive cells and goblet cells (Fig. 12.13) and have a core of connective tissue supporting blood vessels and lymphatic vessels (lacteals). A few smooth muscle cells are also present in villi (Figs 12.10, 12.12 and 12.13) and their contractions move the villi amongst the chyle, thus aiding absorption.

■ *Microvilli.* These are small folds in the apical membrane of each columnar epithelial cell which are revealed by the light microscope as a 'brush border' (Fig. 12.10; see also Fig. 3.4) and which appear as finger-like projections when examined by an electron microscope.

■ *Intestinal glands (crypts of Lieberkühn).* These are tubes which dip into the mucosa as far as the muscularis mucosae (Fig. 12.12). As well as columnar epithelial and goblet cells, Paneth cells (Fig. 12.11), neuroendocrine cells and stem cells (Fig. 12.11) are present in the epithelium of intestinal glands.

The life span of epithelial cells in the mucosa of the small intestine is less than a week; cells at the tip of villi die and are rapidly replaced. It is the mitotic activity (Fig. 12.11) of stem cells in the epithelium at the base of intestinal glands which ensures that new cells are produced. Some of the new cells differentiate and become columnar epithelial cells, others become goblet cells, yet others remain as stem cells. The new columnar and goblet cells migrate from the intestinal glands along the epithelium and up to the tip of the villus where, in turn, they die.

The first part of the small intestine, the duodenum, is characterised by the presence of glands in the submucosal layer (Fig. 12.14). These glands (Brunner's glands) make and secrete alkaline mucus which helps neutralise the acidic

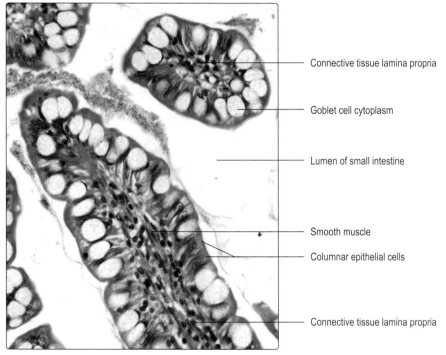

Connective tissue lamina propria

Goblet cell cytoplasm

Lumen of small intestine

Smooth muscle

Columnar epithelial cells

Connective tissue lamina propria

Fig. 12.13 **Small intestine, villi sectioned transversely and longitudinally.** Villi characterise small intestine, and when they are sectioned transversely they appear as islands of cells surrounded by the space of the lumen. (When intestinal glands are sectioned (in large and small intestine) they do not appear as islands of cells.) High magnification.

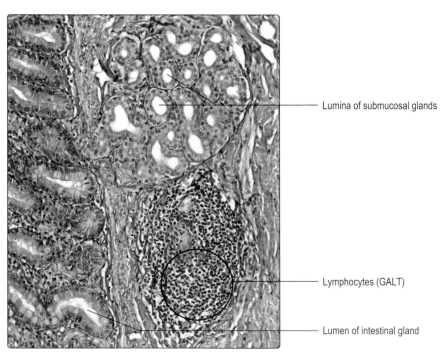

Lumina of submucosal glands

Lymphocytes (GALT)

Lumen of intestinal gland

Fig. 12.14 **Small intestine, duodenum, submucosal (Brunner's) glands, gut (mucosa)-associated lymphoid tissue (GALT) and the base of intestinal glands.** Goblet cell cytoplasm is stained blue/turquoise. Special stain. Low magnification.

chyme entering from the stomach. Secretions from neuroendocrine cells in the duodenum inhibit the action of gastrin and help control the flow of gastric contents to the duodenum.

Within the walls of the small intestine there is a variety of immunocompetent cells, including lymphocytes (mainly T cells), plasma cells (mainly secreting IgA), eosinophils, mast cells and macrophages. Clusters of immune cells (GALT) are present and usually are in the submucosal layer (Fig. 12.14) or the lamina propria. The ileum, however, is characterised by the presence of large accumulations of immune cells which are visible to the unaided eye as white oval-shaped regions. These are known as Peyer's patches. They are present in the lamina propria and may extend into the submucosa and are restricted to the gut wall opposite to the attachment site of the peritoneal membranes.

Large intestine

The large intestine comprises the colon, appendix, rectum and the upper part of the anal canal (Fig. 12.1). Its structure largely conforms to the general plan (Fig. 12.2). The mucosa is similar along the length of the large intestine, and goblet cells (Figs 12.15 and 12.16) are far more common than in the small intestine. The mucosal epithelium dips into the mucosa and forms intestinal glands which reach the muscularis mucosae (Fig. 12.16). This arrangement increases the area of interface between the luminal contents and the epithelial cells. Columnar epithelial cells, absorbing mainly water, are present mainly on or near the luminal surface, and stem cells and a few neuroendocrine cells are also present in the epithelium. Villi and submucosal glands are not present in the large intestine.

The muscularis externa of the large intestine differs from the general plan in that although it has an inner circular layer its outer longitudinal layer is arranged in three bands (taeniae coli). Peristaltic contractions of the muscularis externa move the contents in the lumen towards the anus. Although the large intestine is much shorter than the small intestine, the transit time through the large intestine takes relatively longer at up to about 48 hours. During transit, water and salt absorption occurs and the remnants form feces. The mucus secreted by goblet cells in the epithelium is important in lubricating the movement of feces along the large intestine.

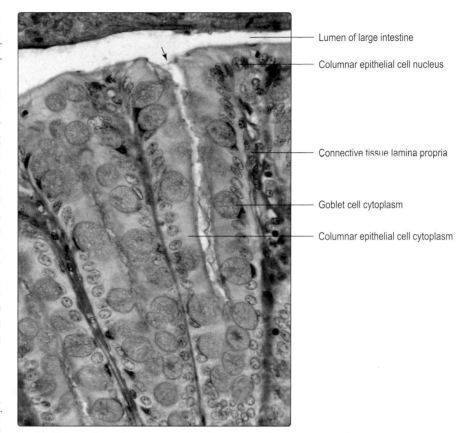

Fig. 12.15 **Large intestine, upper region of intestinal glands.** An arrow shows the entrance to an intestinal gland. Goblet cell cytoplasm is stained blue/turquoise. Special stain. High magnification.

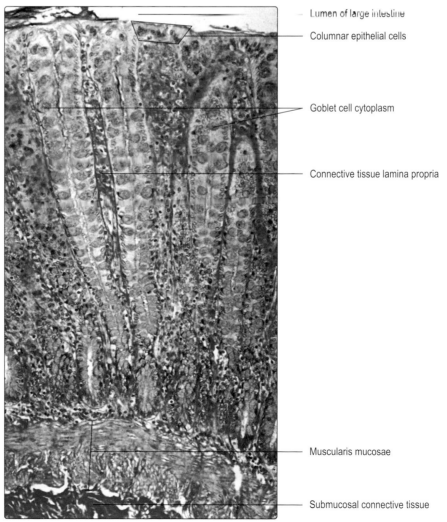

Fig. 12.16 **Large intestine, intestinal glands and muscularis mucosae.** Goblet cell cytoplasm is stained turquoise/blue. Special stain. Low magnification.

Appendix

The appendix is a blind-ended tube connected to the colon. It is similar in structure to the large intestine and lymphoid tissue is a prominent feature (Fig. 12.17). Lymphoid tissue may extend between the muscularis externa and the luminal surface, replacing the submucosa and the mucosa. The lymphoid tissue is most prominent in children, and largely disappears in adulthood as the appendix atrophies.

Liver

The liver is a large, highly vascular, glandular structure situated in the upper abdomen. It has significant roles in the function of the digestive system. It is covered by a connective tissue capsule and, in turn, by peritoneum. The cell type which forms the majority of the parenchyma of the liver is the hepatocyte (Fig. 12.18). The liver receives blood drained from most of the gastrointestinal tract. This brings products of digestion, principally amino acids and monosaccharides, directly from the gut. Hepatocytes synthesise a range of large molecules, some of which they store, e.g. glycogen; others they secrete into blood, e.g. albumin. Hepatocytes also break down absorbed harmful molecules (e.g. alcohol) and waste molecules (e.g. from the breakdown of haemoglobin). Some waste molecules are secreted by hepatocytes into bile (see below), which drains into the duodenum, from where they are eventually excreted in feces.

The liver receives blood from two sources: the hepatic artery, which supplies blood that is high in oxygen content, and the hepatic portal vein, which supplies blood that is low in oxygen content. The hepatic portal vein drains blood from the gastrointestinal tract and carries the molecules produced by digestion to the liver. These two sources of blood pass into liver sinusoids (wide vascular channels) lined by irregularly placed endothelial cells lying on an incomplete basement membrane. Non-migratory macrophages, known as Kupffer cells, are interspersed between the endothelial cells and they phagocytose effete red cells (and microorganisms if present in the blood). Columns of hepatocytes lie alongside the sinusoids separated from the basement membrane by a space (the space of Disse) (Fig. 12.19). Blood passes along the sinusoids and some plasma passes between the endothelial cells into the

space of Disse. The hepatocytes adjacent to the space of Disse take up the small molecules produced by digestion and synthesise larger molecules required by the body. Blood drains from sinusoids into small veins, known as central veins (Fig. 12.18), which join together and leave the liver as the hepatic vein.

Between adjacent hepatocytes there are very small spaces, bile canaliculi (Fig. 12.19). These channels receive bile secreted by hepatocytes. The direction of flow in bile canaliculi is opposite to the blood flow in sinusoids. Bile canaliculi join together and drain into a network of epithelium-lined bile ducts. The bile ducts pass through the liver alongside branches of the hepatic arteries and hepatic portal veins in structures known as portal tracts (Figs 12.18 and 12.20). The ducts join together and eventually bile drains into a single duct which transports bile, via the gall bladder, to the duodenum. Bile aids the digestion of fats as well as being the route by which the breakdown products from the destruction of red blood cells are excreted.

The classical functional unit of the liver is a hexagonal lobule enclosed by connective tissue. In humans, connective tissue is sparse between lobules but is present in portal tracts supporting branches of the hepatic artery, hepatic portal vein and bile duct (Figs 12.18 and 12.20) and around central veins (Fig. 12.18). A fine meshwork of reticulin fibres supports the sinusoids (see Fig. 4.3). From a functional view, it is appropriate to consider the blood supply as

the basis of the functional unit. Hepatocytes closest to where hepatic arteries and hepatic portal veins (in portal tracts) open into sinusoids are exposed to the highest concentrations of oxygen and molecules absorbed from the gut. These include the small molecules produced by digestion and any ingested toxic molecules or harmful microorganisms. Conversely, hepatocytes closest to central veins draining the sinusoids are exposed to lower levels of all these substances. Hepatocytes in different regions may appear similar but, in varying nutritional states and pathological conditions, their appearance may depend on their position in relation to blood supply.

Gall bladder

Ducts draining bile from the liver eventually drain into a single bile duct which drains into the gall bladder. The gall bladder lies on the right, close to the liver, and stores and concentrates bile prior to its release. The gall bladder is lined by a simple columnar epithelium which absorbs fluid and concentrates the bile by up to 20 times. Smooth muscle forms the majority of the wall of the gall bladder and its contraction helps to expel stored bile. Parasympathetic nerves and molecules produced by neuroendocrine cells in the duodenum control the flow of bile in relation to the contents of the gastrointestinal tract. Bile expelled from the gall bladder enters the common bile duct, which drains into the duodenum.

Clinical notes

Chemotherapy Many chemotherapy drugs used to treat cancer target and kill cells in mitosis. As well as killing rapidly dividing cancer cells these drugs kill normal dividing cells such as those in epithelia lining the small (and large) intestine. Normally, intestinal epithelial cells are replaced every few days. After this type of chemotherapy there is impaired replacement of the columnar cells and goblet cells in the intestinal epithelia. As a result, absorption of nutrients and water is impaired and usually diarrhoea occurs.

Appendicitis The appendix is a blind-ended tube which may become inflamed due to stagnation and impaction of the contents of the gut. This results in appendicitis. If the inflammation destroys the wall of the appendix it spreads into the peritoneal cavity. As a result, microorganisms from the gut enter a large potential space where they can readily multiply: this may be fatal.

Fig. 12.17 **Appendix.** Special stain. High magnification.

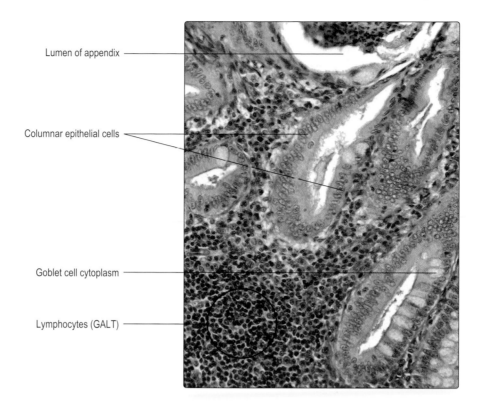

Lumen of appendix —

Columnar epithelial cells —

Goblet cell cytoplasm —

Lymphocytes (GALT) —

Fig. 12.18 **Liver, portal tract and central vein.** The lumen of the artery and the bile duct in the portal tract are very small and difficult to distinguish at this magnification, but the artery is closest to the hepatic portal vein in this figure. Connective tissue is stained green and red blood cells scarlet. Special stain. Very low magnification

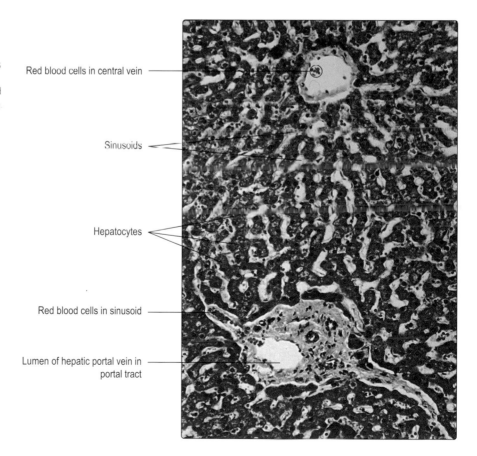

Red blood cells in central vein —

Sinusoids —

Hepatocytes —

Red blood cells in sinusoid —

Lumen of hepatic portal vein in portal tract —

Fig. 12.19 **The arrangement of hepatocytes, sinusoids, the space of Disse and a bile canaliculus.**

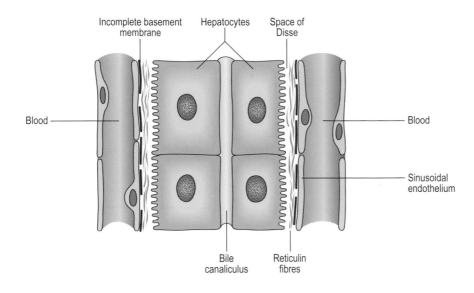

Incomplete basement membrane
Hepatocytes
Space of Disse
Blood
Blood
Sinusoidal endothelium
Bile canaliculus
Reticulin fibres

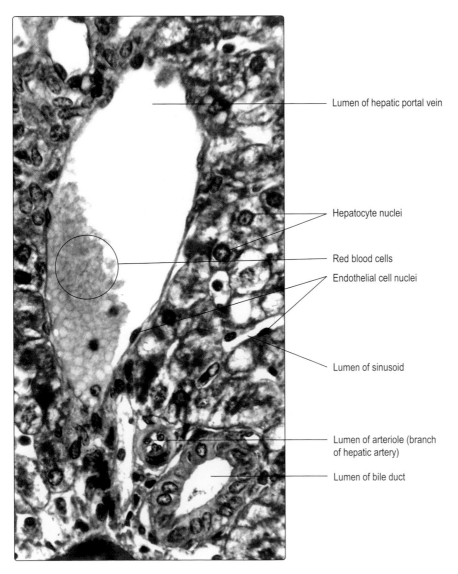

Fig. 12.20 **Liver, portal tract.** Connective tissue and red blood cells are stained blue. Special stain. High magnification.

Lumen of hepatic portal vein

Hepatocyte nuclei

Red blood cells

Endothelial cell nuclei

Lumen of sinusoid

Lumen of arteriole (branch of hepatic artery)

Lumen of bile duct

Pancreas

The pancreas lies in the abdominal cavity and functions as an exocrine and endocrine (Chapter 14) gland. It has a thin connective tissue capsule and is divided into lobules by connective tissue septa. The exocrine cells are columnar epithelial cells (Fig. 12.21) arranged as acini or tubules and they secrete bicarbonate ions (which help neutralise gastric acid) and pancreatic enzymes (proteinases, peptidases, lipases and amylases), which are inactive until they reach the duodenum. The enzymes are stored in zymogen granules in the apical portions of the columnar cells; the nucleus and rough endoplasmic reticulum are in the basal portions of the cells (Fig. 12.21). The release of secretions is controlled by parasympathetic nerves and molecules secreted by neuroendocrine cells in the duodenum. A duct drains each acinus. Ducts join together within the lobules and eventually all join and form a single pancreatic duct. The duct system is lined by epithelial cells which, in the larger ducts, may be a double layer of columnar epithelial cells. The pancreatic duct joins the bile duct and bile and pancreatic juices drain into the duodenum.

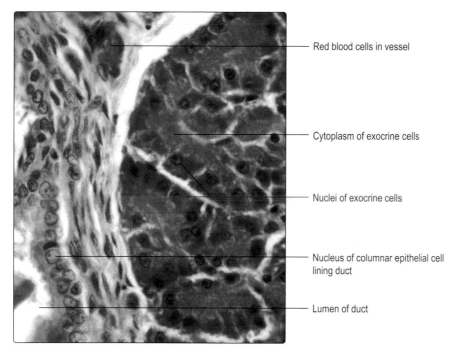

- Red blood cells in vessel
- Cytoplasm of exocrine cells
- Nuclei of exocrine cells
- Nucleus of columnar epithelial cell lining duct
- Lumen of duct

Fig. 12.21 **Pancreas, exocrine cells and part of a duct.** The eosinophilic cytoplasm is due to the proteins in the apical regions of the exocrine cells, and the basal, bluish cytoplasm adjacent to the nuclei and stained with haematoxylin, is due to rough endoplasmic reticulum. High magnification.

Summary

The digestive system
- The digestive system consists of the alimentary canal connecting the mouth to the anus and associated structures, e.g. salivary glands, liver and pancreas.

The alimentary canal
- The alimentary canal has a general pattern of four layers:
  - a mucosa comprising an epithelium, basement membrane, lamina propria and a smooth muscle layer (the muscularis mucosae)
  - a submucosal layer supporting large blood vessels and nerves
  - a muscularis externa comprising an inner circular and an outer longitudinal layer of smooth muscle which contracts and moves the contents of the canal towards the anus
  - an outer covering which is a serosal (peritoneal) membrane in most regions.

Oesophagus
- The oesophagus is lined by a stratified squamous epithelium and has serous and mucous glands in the submucosal layer.
- It has striated voluntary muscle in the muscularis externa in regions close to the mouth and smooth muscle in lower regions.
- It has an outer adventitia binding it to adjacent structures.

Stomach

- The stomach is lined by a simple epithelium. Cells lining gastric pits secrete mucus; cells lining gastric glands (in the main part of the stomach) secrete acid and enzymes.
- It has three layers of smooth muscle in its wall and an outer serosal layer.

Small intestine

- Epithelia covering villi and lining intestinal glands comprise columnar absorptive cells, goblet cells, stem cells and Paneth cells.
- In the duodenum submucosal glands secrete alkaline mucus into the lumen.
- In the ileum lymphoid follicles are usually present.

Large intestine

- A simple epithelium lines intestinal glands and contains absorptive columnar and goblet cells (no villi are present).

Structures associated with the digestive system

- Salivary glands contain serous and mucous cells.
- The tongue is covered by a stratified, squamous epithelium which, on its upper surface, has papillae and taste buds. Mucous and serous glands and lymphoid cells are deep to the epithelium and skeletal muscle forms the inner mass of the tongue.
- The liver is formed mainly of hepatocytes:
  - it receives blood draining most parts of the alimentary canal and synthesises many new molecules and stores glycogen
  - it secretes bile which drains into the duodenum and aids digestion of fats
  - it destroys red blood cells and excretes some waste molecules in bile.
- The pancreas is formed mainly by exocrine cells (endocrine cells are also present):
  - pancreatic enzymes (inactive when secreted) drain into the duodenum, where they begin to digest carbohydrates, proteins and lipids.

Chapter 13
The urinary system

The urinary system consists of paired kidneys and the urinary tract, which comprises paired ureters, a urinary bladder and a urethra (Fig. 13.1). Urine is produced by the kidneys and passes along the ureters to the urinary bladder, where it is stored until it is voided via the urethra. The route taken by urine along the urethra to the exterior is an independent closed system in females, but is shared with the reproductive system in males (Chapter 15).

The urinary system is essential in maintaining the homeostasis of the body. It does this by regulating the water and mineral salts in, and the acid–base balance of, blood. It is particularly important in excreting toxic molecules containing nitrogen (e.g. urea and creatinine) produced by the breakdown of endogenous proteins. The urinary system also ensures that useful molecules in blood, e.g. proteins and carbohydrates, are not lost during the formation of urine. The toxic molecules and excess ions, dissolved in water, leave the kidneys as urine, which passes along the urinary tract before being voided at micturition. In addition, the kidneys produce and secrete into blood two molecules, renin and erythropoietin. The former is important in regulating blood pressure and the latter in stimulating the formation of red blood cells.

Kidneys

The gross structure of a kidney is best described as seen in a longitudinal hemi-section (Fig. 13.2). Facing towards the mid-line of the body, each kidney has an indentation forming a hilum. At the hilum blood enters and leaves each kidney in, respectively, a renal artery and a renal vein, and urine drains into a ureter.

The gross appearance of the kidney displays an outer and an inner region, the cortex and the medulla. The cortex has a granular appearance due to the presence of spherical structures about 200 µm in diameter known as renal corpuscles. These corpuscles filter blood in the initial stage in the formation of urine. The cortex also contains convoluted tubules involved in forming urine. Renal corpuscles are not present in the medulla and the medulla appears smooth or may show striations. Straight and arching tubules are present in the medulla and they also are involved in forming urine. Renal corpuscles and tubules may be distinguished in histological sections even at low magnification (Fig. 13.3). In humans, the medulla projects centrally as several pyramids and the cortex extends as columns between the pyramids (Fig. 13.2). The apices of the pyramids project as renal papillae into urine-filled spaces (minor calyces). Urine drains from tubules in the medulla into the calyces. Each minor calyx drains urine into major calyces that together form the renal pelvis. The relatively large, fluid filled space of each renal pelvis drains into a ureter (Fig. 13.2). Fat cells surround the renal pelvis, the ureter and vessels at the hilum of the kidney and pack a space known as the renal sinus. A dense layer of fat surrounds each kidney.

The blood supply to kidneys ensures that the whole volume of blood in the body passes through the kidneys every 5 minutes or so. The arrangement of blood vessels is based on supplying (and draining) each medullary pyramid and its associated cortical tissues separately, a unit described as a renal lobe. (The human kidney is multilobar, but unilobar kidneys occur in many species.) Each renal artery branches and forms interlobar arteries. In turn, interlobar

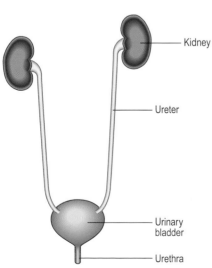

Fig. 13.1 **The components of the urinary tract.**

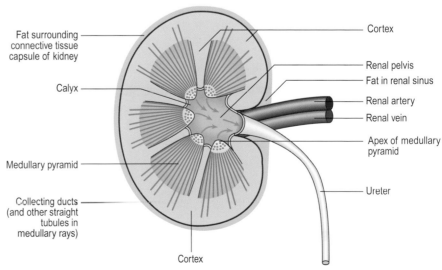

Fig. 13.2 **A longitudinal section through a kidney.** Arrows show the direction of flow of urine.

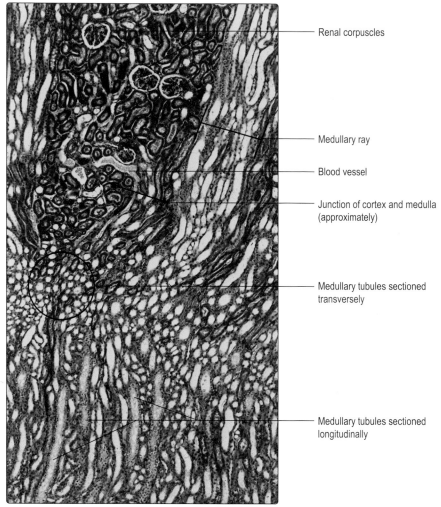

Renal corpuscles

Medullary ray

Blood vessel

Junction of cortex and medulla
(approximately)

Medullary tubules sectioned
transversely

Medullary tubules sectioned
longitudinally

Fig. 13.3 **Kidney, cortex and medulla.** The approximate junction between the cortex and medulla is shown (renal corpuscles are not present in the medulla). Connective tissue is sparse and stained blue. Special stain. Very low magnification.

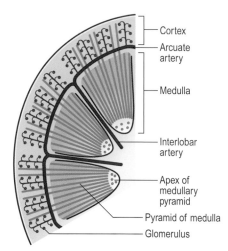

Cortex

Arcuate
artery

Medulla

Interlobar
artery

Apex of
medullary
pyramid

Pyramid of medulla

Glomerulus

Fig. 13.4 **The arrangement of arteries supplying glomeruli in the kidney.**

arteries branch further and then form arcuate arteries which arch between the cortex and medulla (Fig. 13.4). Branches from arcuate arteries eventually supply each renal corpuscle with an afferent arteriole. This arrangement is essential in filtering the blood (see below) as well as supplying oxygen and nutrients.

Each afferent arteriole divides within a renal corpuscle into capillaries, known as glomerular capillaries (Fig. 13.5), and these drain from the corpuscle into an efferent arteriole (Fig. 13.6). This arrangement of capillaries draining to an arteriole is unique to the kidney and results in a relatively high blood pressure in glomerular capillaries (Fig. 13.5) which aids the filtration of blood. Efferent arterioles divide and form a second network of capillaries. Some of these capillaries are straight vessels, vasa recta, which lie between straight tubules in the kidney whereas others form an extensive meshwork surrounding convoluted tubules in the cortex (Fig. 13.6). The second set of capillaries supplies oxygen and nutrients to the cells of the kidney and is also involved in modifying the filtrate and forming urine. Veins drain capillaries (other than glomerular capillaries) in the kidney and the routes they take closely follow the arterial pattern.

Nephrons and collecting ducts

A nephron is the functional unit of the kidney (Fig. 13.6) and there are about a million in each kidney in humans. A nephron consists of a renal corpuscle, which filters blood, and the uriniferous tubule attached to it which drains and modifies the filtrate. Eventually, the modified filtrate becomes urine and drains, via collecting ducts, into the renal pelvis.

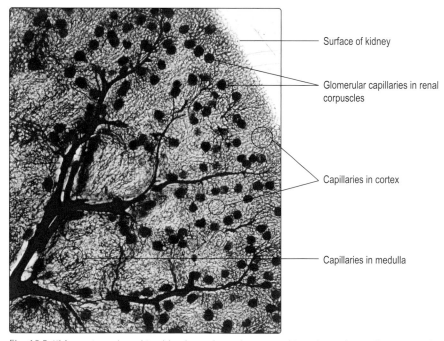

Surface of kidney

Glomerular capillaries in renal
corpuscles

Capillaries in cortex

Capillaries in medulla

Fig. 13.5 **Kidney.** Large branching blood vessels are shown supplying glomerular capillaries in renal corpuscles in the cortex. The network of capillaries in the cortex and medulla is also displayed. Special procedure showing blood vessels. Very low magnification.

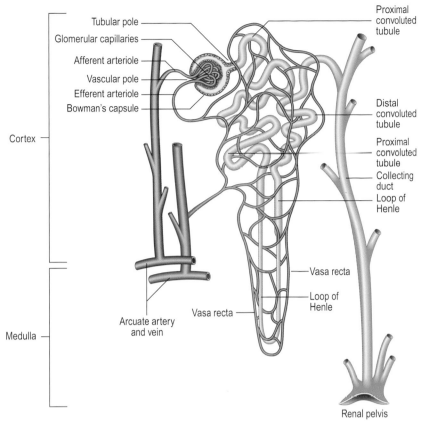

Fig. 13.6 **The structure of a nephron (renal corpuscle and uriniferous tubule) and related blood vessels.**

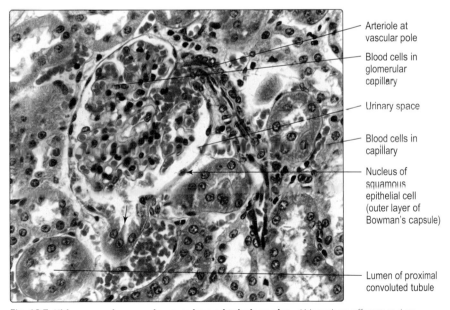

Fig. 13.7 **Kidney, renal corpuscle, vascular and tubular poles.** Although an afferent and an efferent artery, respectively, supply and drain glomerular capillaries via the vascular pole, only one arteriole is apparent in this section. The arrow shows the tubular pole where filtrate in the urinary space drains into the proximal tubule. High magnification.

Renal corpuscles

Each renal corpuscle consists of glomerular capillaries (a renal glomerulus) (Fig. 13.5) within a Bowman's capsule. The capsule is shaped like a hollow, double-walled cup (Fig. 13.6) and it is lined by epithelial cells. The outer parietal layer of Bowman's capsule is lined by squamous epithelial cells (Fig. 13.7) and it is continuous with the inner visceral layer of epithelial cells. The cells of the inner layer, known as podocytes, have numerous cytoplasmic processes which abut the capillaries of the glomerulus. The endothelial cells lining the capillaries and the podocytes (and their fused basement membranes) form the filtration barrier between the blood and the filtrate. The space between the inner and outer layers of the capsule receives the filtrate and is known as the urinary space (Fig. 13.7) even though the filtrate is not yet urine.

Each Bowman's capsule has two poles, and it is extremely rare to see all the features of each pole in any one (histological) section of a corpuscle.

- *Vascular pole* (Figs 13.6 and 13.7). At this pole an afferent arteriole enters each renal corpuscle, branches and forms glomerular capillaries. These capillaries rejoin and drain into an efferent arteriole (not a venule), which leaves the corpuscle at the vascular pole.
- *Tubular pole* (Figs 13.6–13.8). At this pole the filtrate drains from the urinary space of the renal corpuscle. It enters the proximal part of the uriniferous tubule, which extends from the parietal layer of Bowman's capsule at this pole.

Filtration

Blood in glomerular capillaries is filtered through the endothelium lining the capillaries. It then traverses the fused basement membranes of the endothelium and of the adjacent podocytes (the visceral epithelial cells of Bowman's capsule) (Fig. 13.9).

Filtration is affected by:

- the pressure of blood in the afferent arteriole
- the pressure of blood in the efferent arteriole; this provides resistance to the outflow of blood from the glomerular capillaries causing a relatively high pressure in the glomerular capillaries
- fenestrations in the endothelium of the glomerular capillaries; these fenestrations retain molecules over about 69 000 daltons in the blood (e.g. albumin)
- the fused basement membranes; these are charged and repel many protein molecules
- the structure of the podocytes. Podocytes have numerous large and small cytoplasmic foot processes (Figs 13.9 and 13.10). The smaller foot processes abut the basement membrane and there are small spaces between them. It is probable that this arrangement of the foot processes is involved in preventing some proteins from passing from blood into the filtrate.

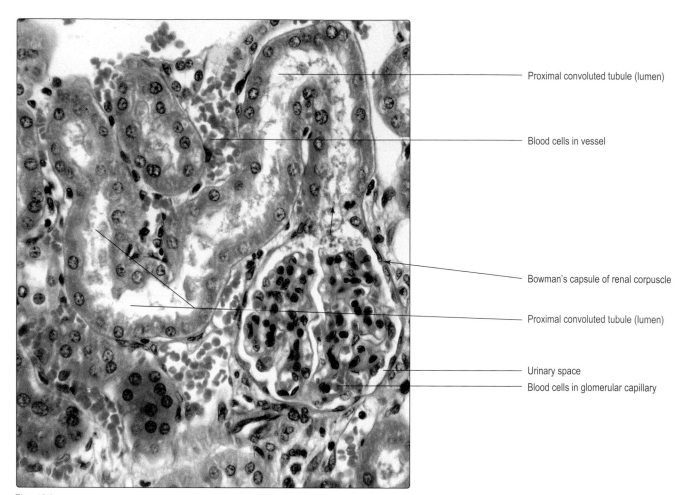

Proximal convoluted tubule (lumen)

Blood cells in vessel

Bowman's capsule of renal corpuscle

Proximal convoluted tubule (lumen)

Urinary space

Blood cells in glomerular capillary

Fig. 13.8 **Kidney, renal corpuscle, tubular pole and the initial part of the draining proximal tubule.** The arrow shows the tubular pole where filtrate from the urinary space drains into the proximal tubule. This section along some of the length of the proximal tubule displays the first part of its convoluted course, in the plane of the section. The vascular pole of the corpuscle is not in the plane of this section. High magnification.

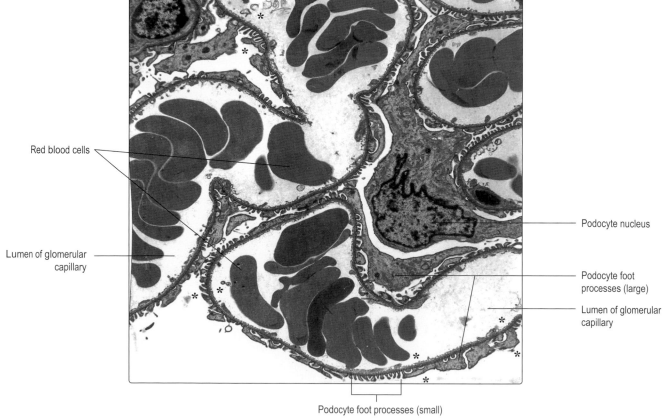

Red blood cells

Lumen of glomerular capillary

Podocyte nucleus

Podocyte foot processes (large)

Lumen of glomerular capillary

Podocyte foot processes (small)

Fig. 13.9 **Kidney, podocytes and glomerular capillaries.** Electron micrograph. The filtration barrier between blood in glomerular capillaries and the urinary space which drains the filtrate is thin. The complexity and the size of the cytoplasmic foot processes of podocytes adjacent to the outer wall of the capillaries are shown. Some regions of the filtration barrier are shown between asterisks. Low magnification.

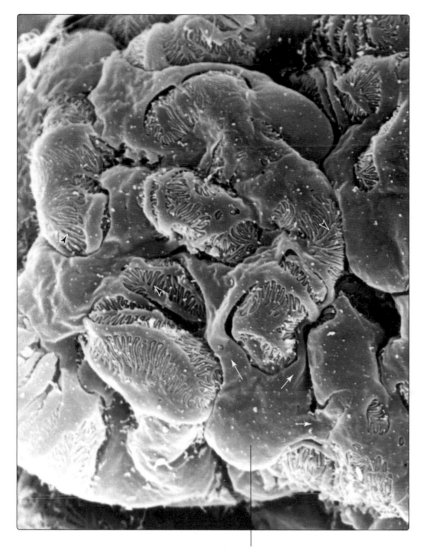

Podocyte showing three foot processes (large)

Fig. 13.10 **Kidney, podocytes.** Electron micrograph. This scanning view looks at podocytes as though from the urinary space. Arrows (white) indicate large cytoplasmic processes extending from one podocyte. Numerous smaller cytoplasmic processes (arrowheads) wrap around the glomerular capillaries. Low magnification.

of the sodium and chloride ions. This resorption is facilitated by microvilli on the apical (luminal) surfaces of the epithelial cells lining the proximal tubules, providing a large interface between the cell membrane and the filtrate. The movement of sodium ions out of the filtrate is an energy-dependent process powered by mitochondria in the epithelial cells. Water passively follows the sodium ions.

Resorbed water and ions readily pass into blood in the capillaries, which form a meshwork around proximal convoluted tubules (Figs 13.7, 13.8 and 13.11). The movement of these ions and water helps maintain electrical neutrality and osmotic equilibrium in the capillaries. Amino acids and glucose in the glomerular filtrate are resorbed from the filtrate in proximal tubules and return to blood. Small proteins in the filtrate are taken into the epithelial cells lining proximal tubules by endocytosis. After fusion of the endocytotic vesicles with lysosomes the proteins are digested and the amino acids produced return to blood.

In addition, the epithelial cells lining proximal tubules (in humans) are able to secrete waste molecules such as creatinine into the lumen of the proximal tubules, and they are able to prevent the resorption of some toxins and drugs which have passed from blood into the glomerular filtrate.

Loop of Henle

The tubule of the first part of a loop of Henle drains a proximal convoluted tubule and it passes (descends) as a straight tubule towards, and usually into, the medulla. The tubule then loops and passes (ascends) as a straight tubule into the cortex (Fig. 13.6). The lower part of the descending limb of the loop of Henle and some of the ascending limb are tubules that have relatively wide lumina and thin walls. These 'thin' regions are lined by a simple squamous epithelium (Fig. 13.12). The final portion of the loop of Henle is lined by a simple cuboidal epithelium and it continues, in the cortex, as a distal convoluted tubule which is lined by a similar cuboidal epithelium.

The functions of the various regions of loops of Henle are related to producing a hypertonic environment in the sparse connective tissue (interstitium) between tubules in the medulla (Fig. 13.3). This is essential for the production of hypertonic urine (see below). The interstitium comprises few cells, e.g. fibroblasts, sparse fibres and complex

The filtrate passing out of blood and into the urinary space of Bowman's capsule is known as the glomerular filtrate and it flows at a rate of about 190 litres/day, of which 188.5 litres is reabsorbed as it passes along the uriniferous tubules and collecting ducts. As a result approximately 1.5 litres of urine are excreted per day.

Uriniferous tubule

Each uriniferous tubule drains the filtrate from the urinary space of a Bowman's capsule (Fig. 13.6). The filtrate enters the proximal convoluted tubule, the first part of the uriniferous tubule, and this takes a coiled course in the cortex before straightening. This straight tubule continues and forms a loop (the loop of Henle), which extends from the cortex towards the medulla; many loops of Henle extend deep into the medulla. Each loop of Henle returns to the cortex

and continues as a distal convoluted tubule which eventually drains into a straight collecting duct in the cortex (Fig. 13.6). (Collecting ducts are not usually described as part of the nephron.)

Proximal convoluted tubule

Proximal convoluted tubules are longer than distal convoluted tubules and thus are the predominant tubule seen in histological sections of the kidney cortex (Fig. 13.11). They are lined by simple cuboidal (or low columnar) epithelial cells (Figs 13.7 and 13.8). The lumen of proximal tubules is indistinct in many histological sections as the lumen that transports filtrate in life is virtually filled by the apical surface of the epithelial cells.

Proximal convoluted tubules resorb about 80% of the water that has passed into the glomerular filtrate and many carbohydrate molecules. Several factors are involved in modulating the tonicity of the interstitium:

- the descending thin limb of the loop of Henle is freely permeable to sodium and chloride ions and water
- the majority of the (cuboidal) epithelial cells lining the ascending limb is impermeable to water
- cuboidal epithelial cells lining the ascending limb actively pump sodium ions into the interstitium and chloride ions follow passively; the hormone aldosterone from the adrenal glands (Chapter 14) stimulates this resorption of sodium ions
- some ions in the interstitium diffuse into nearby straight capillaries (vasa recta) (Fig. 13.12)
- some ions re-enter the descending limb but may be pumped out again as they pass again along the distal (ascending) limb
- the net movement of ions results in:
  - a hypertonic interstitium (particularly near the apex of the medullary pyramids)
  - a hypotonic fluid passing into the distal tubule in the cortex.

The term 'countercurrent multiplier mechanism' is used to describe this complex movement of ions.

Distal convoluted tubule

Distal convoluted tubules are shorter than proximal convoluted tubules so appear to be fewer in number in histological sections (Fig. 13.11). They are lined by a simple epithelium consisting of small cuboidal or low columnar cells (Fig. 13.13) which do not have microvilli. As a result, in comparison with proximal tubules, distal tubules appear to have more distinct lumina and more closely packed cells in their walls (Fig. 13.13).

Each distal convoluted tubule returns to the vascular pole of the renal corpuscle from which it arose and forms part of a functional unit known as the juxtaglomerular apparatus (see below). Epithelial cells lining distal tubules resorb sodium ions from the filtrate. Resorbed molecules return to blood in nearby capillaries (Fig. 13.11). In addition, hydrogen ions are secreted. The ion movements in this region are important in regulating the tonicity and acid–base balance of blood. The movements of these ions are affected by the hormone aldosterone from the adrenal gland (Chapter 14).

Collecting ducts

Several distal convoluted tubules in the cortex drain into each collecting duct (Fig. 13.6). Collecting ducts are straight tubules which lie clustered in parallel with other straight tubules (e.g. loops of Henle) that pass between the cortex and the medulla. The regions containing parallel tubules are known as medullary rays (Fig. 13.3). Collecting ducts are lined by a simple cuboidal epithelium and in the medulla are surrounded by the hypertonic interstitium. This aids resorption of water and the production of hypertonic urine. Two hormones are involved in controlling this resorption of water and some ions. Aldosterone stimulates the epithelial cells lining collecting ducts to resorb sodium and chloride ions, and water follows passively. In addition, antidiuretic hormone (from

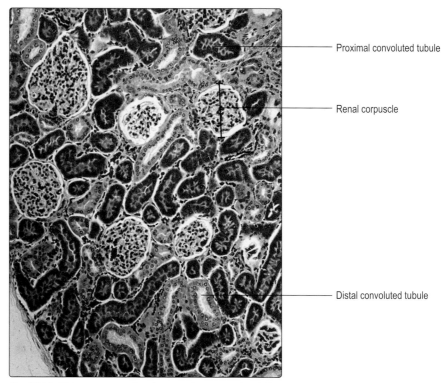

Fig. 13.11 **Kidney, cortex.** Renal corpuscles, proximal and distal convoluted tubules. This stain shows red blood cells as scarlet and their location is readily seen even at this low magnification. Special stain. Low magnification.

Proximal convoluted tubule

Renal corpuscle

Distal convoluted tubule

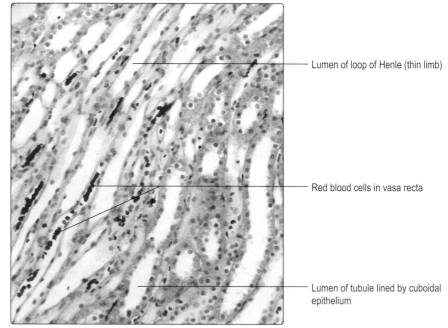

Fig. 13.12 **Kidney, medulla, vasa recta and tubules sectioned along their length.** This stain shows red blood cells as scarlet. Special stain. Medium magnification.

Lumen of loop of Henle (thin limb)

Red blood cells in vasa recta

Lumen of tubule lined by cuboidal epithelium

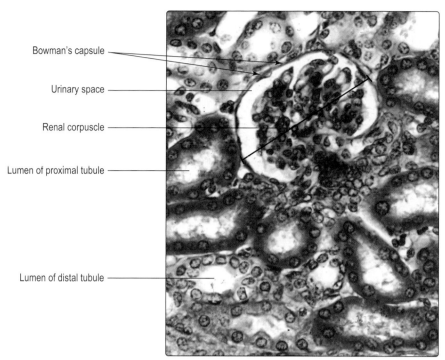

Fig. 13.13 **Kidney, cortex.** Connective tissue is stained blue. Special stain. High magnification.

- Bowman's capsule
- Urinary space
- Renal corpuscle
- Lumen of proximal tubule
- Lumen of distal tubule

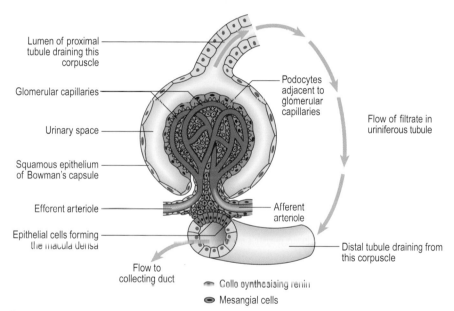

- Lumen of proximal tubule draining this corpuscle
- Glomerular capillaries
- Urinary space
- Squamous epithelium of Bowman's capsule
- Efferent arteriole
- Epithelial cells forming the macula densa
- Flow to collecting duct
- Podocytes adjacent to glomerular capillaries
- Flow of filtrate in uriniferous tubule
- Afferent arteriole
- Distal tubule draining from this corpuscle
- Cells synthesising renin
- Mesangial cells

Fig. 13.14 **The juxtaglomerular apparatus.** Arrows indicate direction of flow of filtrate.

(Figs 13.14 and 13.15). These epithelial cells probably detect changes in sodium concentration in the filtrate from that corpuscle and help control the rate of filtration by affecting renin secretion.

Connective tissue within, and adjacent to, the renal corpuscle is known as mesangial tissue and it is sparse. Mesangial cells around glomerular capillaries and in the region of the juxtaglomerular apparatus are able to contract and may affect blood flow in the region. In addition, they have phagocytic functions which may be involved in maintaining the basement membranes filtering the blood. Erythropoietin, a molecule which stimulates the production of red cells by bone marrow, is produced by kidneys and it is possible that mesangial cells are the source of this hormone.

Urinary tract

Renal pelves and ureters

Urine drains from the ducts of Bellini in the medulla of each kidney into the lumen of the pelvis of the kidney. The renal pelves are lined by transitional epithelium, the specialised layered epithelium (urothelium) lining all the urinary tract. Each pelvis narrows and is continuous with a ureter (Fig. 13.2).

The wall of each ureter is formed from three layers (Fig. 13.16):

- *An inner lining mucosa.* The mucosa comprises the transitional epithelium lining the lumen and the underlying, supporting connective tissue. This specialised epithelium prevents excess ions and toxic molecules in hypertonic urine from diffusing from the urine through the epithelium and returning to circulate in blood.
- *A middle muscularis layer.* The muscularis is composed of an outer longitudinal and an inner circular layer of smooth muscle in the upper two-thirds of the ureter. In the lower third, there is an additional outer layer of smooth muscle that spirals around the long axis of the ureter. The muscularis layer undergoes peristaltic contractions and propels urine along the ureter towards and into the bladder.
- *A thin connective tissue covering.* The outer connective tissue covering holds each ureter against the adjacent posterior abdominal wall and separates them from overlying peritoneum (the serous membrane of the peritoneal cavity).

the posterior pituitary gland; see Chapter 14) controls the permeability of the cells lining collecting ducts and regulates the amount of water lost in urine. Collecting ducts join together and form wider ducts (of Bellini) which drain the urine into minor calyces at the medullary papillae, and thence into the major calyces of the renal pelvis.

Juxtaglomerular apparatus

Each juxtaglomerular apparatus (Fig. 13.14) involves an afferent arteriole supplying blood to glomerular capillaries in a renal corpuscle, the efferent arteriole draining these capillaries and adjacent connective tissue. In addition, a short region of the distal tubule of the uriniferous tubule draining filtrate from that corpuscle and lying adjacent to the vascular pole, is also involved in the juxtaglomerular apparatus.

Cells in the wall of afferent arterioles secrete the hormone renin. Via its effects on the liver and lungs, renin controls the production of a molecule (angiotensin) which in turn stimulates the production of aldosterone by the adrenal glands (Chapter 14). The epithelial cells lining the distal tubule at the vascular pole appear to be packed together. This region is known as the macula densa

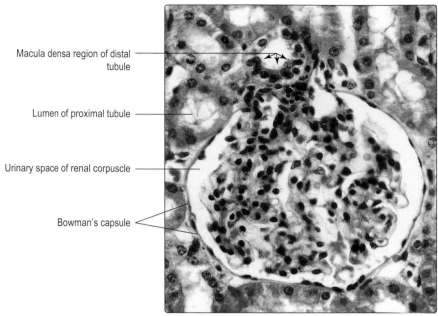

Macula densa region of distal tubule

Lumen of proximal tubule

Urinary space of renal corpuscle

Bowman's capsule

Fig. 13.15 **Kidney, cortex, renal corpuscle, macula densa of the distal tubule.** High magnification.

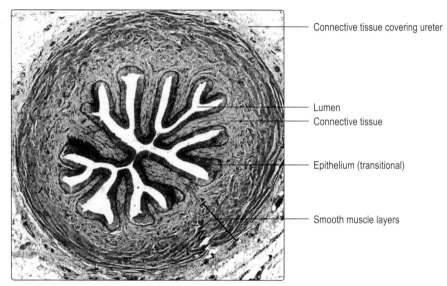

Connective tissue covering ureter

Lumen
Connective tissue

Epithelium (transitional)

Smooth muscle layers

Fig. 13.16 **Ureter, transverse section.** Connective tissue is stained green. Special stain. Very low magnification.

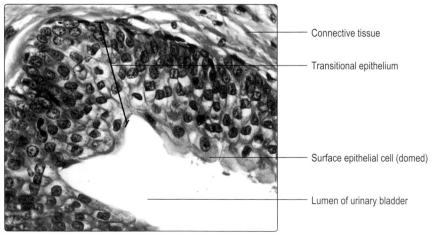

Connective tissue

Transitional epithelium

Surface epithelial cell (domed)

Lumen of urinary bladder

Fig. 13.17 **Bladder, mucosa.** High magnification.

Urine drains along each ureter and into the urinary bladder. Both ureters pass obliquely through the wall of the bladder and this helps prevent back flow of urine into the ureter

Urinary bladder

The urinary bladder is similar to the ureters in that its wall comprises three layers: a mucosa, a muscularis and an outer layer. However, the bladder is able to distend and store large quantities of urine and, after infancy, it is able to contract and expel urine at socially acceptable times.

The bladder mucosa is composed of transitional epithelium (urothelium) and a supporting connective tissue lamina propria (Fig. 13.17). The mucosa is folded and forms rugae in an empty bladder and there are several layers of cells in the epithelium; some surface cells may appear domed (Fig. 13.17). In addition, in the empty bladder parts of the cell membrane of surface epithelial cells are drawn into the cytoplasm. As the volume of urine stored in the bladder increases the rugae unfold, the number of cell layers in the epithelium decreases and the epithelial cells are flattened and their cell membranes lengthen. The epithelium lining the bladder is impermeable and it ensures that hypertonic urine does not equilibrate with surrounding isotonic tissues and blood, and that toxic molecules, e.g. urea, remain in urine and are excreted.

The lamina propria of the bladder mucosa connects the epithelium to the muscularis layer, which is known as the detrusor muscle. The smooth muscle cells in the detrusor muscle are arranged in three interlacing layers. Contraction of the detrusor muscle is brought about by stimulation of the muscle cells by parasympathetic nerves which are under conscious control after infancy. This contraction empties the bladder as urine is voided via the urethra. Parts of the bladder are covered by peritoneum and, as the bladder fills, it moves smoothly against adjacent structures. Connective tissue over other parts of the bladder attaches it to adjacent structures.

Urethra

The urethra is a tube that carries urine from the urinary bladder to the exterior. In the male, it also shares reproductive functions. Further details of the male urethra are given in Chapter 15. In females, the urethra is a relatively short tube and most is lined with a stratified squamous epithelium.

Clinical note

Glomerular disease An abnormally thickened basement membrane between the endothelial cells lining the glomerular capillaries and the podocytes causes one type of glomerular disease. Usually, the thickened basement membrane allows molecules which are normally retained in the blood to pass through the membrane and into the filtrate. Albumin normally is too big to pass into the filtrate but in glomerular disease it passes through in such large quantities that it is not resorbed fully and thus appears in the urine. One cause of thickening of the basement membrane is the deposition of circulating antigen–antibody complexes on the membrane.

Clinical note

Bladder cancer Carcinogens (cancer-causing substances) are widely used in chemical industries, particularly in those producing dyes and rubber. Without due care, people working in these industries are at increased risk of developing bladder cancer. The carcinogens and/or their metabolites are excreted via the kidneys, and the bladder epithelium, exposed to high levels of the carcinogens, undergoes cancerous changes.

Summary

The urinary system
- This consists of paired kidneys and the urinary tract (paired ureters, urinary bladder and urethra).

Kidneys
- The kidneys comprise cortex and medulla.
- The functional unit is the nephron, comprising the renal corpuscle and uriniferous tubule.
- Renal corpuscles are present in the cortex:
  - an afferent arteriole supplies glomerular capillaries within each corpuscle and an efferent arteriole drains the glomerular capillaries
  - the glomerular capillaries are surrounded by a double-walled cup lined by epithelial cells
  - the inner layer of epithelial cells (podocytes) is closely applied to the endothelial cells lining the capillaries and they share basement membranes:
    - filtration of blood occurs across the endothelial cells, basement membranes and podocytes
    - the filtrate enters the urinary space between the walls of the cup
    - the filtrate drains from the cup into a uriniferous tubule.
- Each uriniferous tubule comprises an initial, convoluted proximal tubule (in the cortex), a straight looped portion (loop of Henle) extending from the cortex and into the medulla and a distal convoluted tubule (in the cortex).
- The low columnar epithelial cells lining proximal tubules absorb water, proteins and many of the filtered sodium and chloride ions.
- Some of the cuboidal epithelial cells lining the loops of Henle actively pump sodium ions into the surrounding connective tissue, which becomes hypertonic.
- Cuboidal epithelial cells lining the distal tubules resorb sodium ions.
- Some resorbed ions return to blood capillaries in the cortex and medulla.
- Uriniferous tubules drain into collecting ducts.
- Aldosterone and antidiuretic hormone control the amount of water and ions resorbed and the tonicity of urine, thus aiding homeostasis.

Ureters
- Each transports urine from a renal pelvis to the urinary bladder.
- They are lined by a mucosa consisting of a transitional (multilayered) epithelium and connective tissue:
  - the transitional epithelium ensures hypertonic urine does not equilibrate with isotonic tissue fluid and blood
- They have smooth muscle layers which contract and pass the urine into the bladder.
- They are attached by an outer layer of connective tissue to adjacent structures.

Urinary bladder
- The urinary bladder has a mucosa and muscularis similar to the ureter but is able to store a large volume of urine. As urine is stored the mucosa unfolds, the number of layers of epithelial cells is reduced and the epithelial cells flatten.
- After infancy, parasympathetic nerves (under conscious control) stimulate contraction of the muscularis and this empties the bladder into the urethra at micturition.

Urethra
- It is short in females and lined by a stratified squamous epithelium.
- It is longer in males and shared with the reproductive system.

Chapter 14
The endocrine system

The endocrine system comprises cells which synthesise particular molecules and secrete them into blood vessels. This contrasts with exocrine secretions in which secreted molecules pass along a duct system to their site of action, e.g. from salivary glands to the mouth. The particular molecules secreted by endocrine cells are known as hormones and the vascular circulation carries them around the body where they interact with various cells described as target cells. The principal means by which hormones achieve their specific action is by interacting with receptor molecules expressed by the target cells in various tissues and organs. Once stimulated, target cells respond in a variety of ways, e.g. by increasing synthesis of certain molecules. Hormones may be steroids, peptides or proteins, or other molecules derived from amino acids. In general, hormones are involved in regulating metabolic activities in cells in many organs and tissues of the body, many of which are important in controlling homeostasis.

The endocrine organs comprise the pituitary gland, thyroid gland, parathyroid glands, adrenal (suprarenal) glands and the pineal gland. In addition, the pancreas contains clusters of endocrine cells known as islets of Langerhans amongst the pancreatic exocrine cells (Chapter 12), the gonads contain cells secreting reproductive hormones (Chapters 15 and 16) and secretions from endocrine cells in the hypothalamus affect the secretory activities of the pituitary gland (see below). There are also small groups of neuroendocrine cells in many other regions, e.g. in the epithelial linings of the gastrointestinal tract. Some are known as paracrine cells and their secretions act in surrounding areas.

All endocrine glands and endocrine cells are well supplied by blood providing the metabolites needed to synthesise hormones. The capillaries in endocrine glands are fenestrated and most hormones are secreted directly into them. A fine meshwork of reticulin fibres supports most endocrine cells and capillaries in endocrine glands. This arrangement facilitates the movement of molecules from and to the capillaries.

Hypothalamus and pituitary gland (hypophysis)

The hypothalamus and pituitary gland function together (Fig. 14.1). The hypothalamus is the part of the brain connected by a stalk to the pituitary gland. The hormones produced by the hypothalamus and the pituitary affect the function of many cells in different parts of the body.

The pituitary gland is situated in the cranial cavity in a depression in the sphenoid bone of the skull known as the pituitary fossa. The pituitary has a secretory (glandular) and a neural component called, respectively, the adenohypophysis and neurohypophysis. Connective tissue surrounds these two components as a capsule. The components differ in embryological origin,

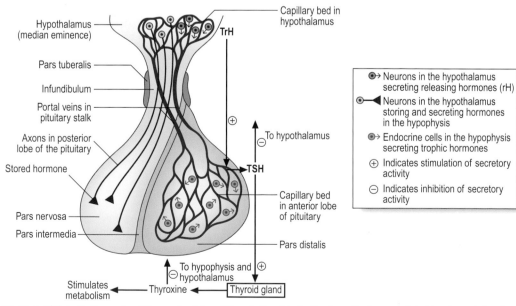

Fig. 14.1 **The structure of the pituitary gland (hypophysis) and its relationship to the hypothalamus.** Only blood vessels involved in the portal circulation are shown. An example of how feedback mechanisms affect the production of thyroid-releasing hormone (TrH) from the hypothalamus, thyroid-stimulating hormone (TSH) from the pituitary gland, and thyroxine from the thyroid gland is shown.

structure and function. The adenohypophysis develops from oral ectoderm and it has clusters or strands of secretory (glandular) cells. The neurohypophysis develops from the part of the brain which forms the hypothalamus. Nerve axons are a prominent structural component of the neurohypophysis and hormones are released from the axons.

The hormones secreted by the pituitary gland are dependent in two distinct ways on hormones produced by cells in the hypothalamus (Fig. 14.1).

- *Adenohypophysis and its vascular connections* (Fig. 14.1). A portal system of capillaries connects the hypothalamus, via the pituitary stalk, with the adenohypophysis. (The definition of a portal system is two capillary beds connected by a set of veins; see hepatic portal system Chapters 10 and 12.) Some hormones produced by neurons in the hypothalamus are secreted into the first capillary bed in the hypothalamus. These capillaries drain into portal veins which carry the hormones along the pituitary stalk to the second capillary bed in the adenohypophysis. By this route hormones from the hypothalamus interact specifically with endocrine cells in the adenohypophysis and control their secretion of a variety of other hormones.

  The hypothalamic hormones which pass in the portal system to the adenohypophysis are peptides and most stimulate specific cells in the adenohypophysis to release their specific hormone. These hypothalamic peptides are known as releasing hormones (rH). For example, the rH from the hypothalamus that stimulates cells in the adenohypophysis to release their hormone which stimulates the thyroid is known as thyroid-releasing hormone (TrH). The pituitary hormone is known as thyroid-stimulating hormone (TSH) and it stimulates the thyroid gland to secrete thyroid hormones, e.g. thyroxine (Fig. 14.1). (In contrast, a few peptide hormones from the hypothalamus inhibit the release of some hormones from the adenohypophysis.)

- *Neurohypophysis and its neural connections* (Fig. 14.1). Axonal processes of some nerve cell bodies in the hypothalamus extend along the pituitary stalk and into the part

of the pituitary gland formed by the neurohypophysis. These neurons synthesise peptide hormones which pass along their axons. These hormones are stored in the end regions of the axons in the neurohypophysis before they are released into the vascular system.

Adenohypophysis

The adenohypophysis consists of three parts, the pars distalis (anterior lobe), the pars intermedia and the pars tuberalis (Fig. 14.1). The cells of the pars distalis form several specific hormones (see below). In humans, the pars intermedia and pars tuberalis are relatively small regions and their significance is not clear.

The cells of the pars distalis have been categorised by the reaction of their cytoplasm to various dyes. Cells that bind dyes are termed chromophils and those that do not are categorised as chromophobes. In routine H&E preparations some chromophils bind eosin and are known as acidophils; others bind haematoxylin and are known as basophils (Fig. 14.2). The differences are due to variations in the pH of the hormones stored as cytoplasmic granules in the

endocrine cells. The cytoplasm of chromophobes is virtually unstained with most dyes, and in some chromophobes the cytoplasm is sparse (Fig. 14.3). Other methods of staining cells of the pars distalis emphasise the differences between the chemical composition of their cells by specifically staining the glycoproteins in basophils (Fig. 14.3). Immunohistochemical methods using light and electron microscopy have now determined precisely which cells in the pars distalis produce the various anterior lobe hormones.

Hormones produced by the adenohypophysis are collectively termed trophic hormones in that they stimulate the release of other hormones from endocrine cells in endocrine glands or in other regions. In general, each endocrine cell in the pars distalis produces only one type of trophic hormone. Some acidophils produce the protein somatotrophin, which is also known as growth hormone (GH) as it is important in stimulating growth, particularly in bones. Other acidophils produce the protein prolactin (PrL), a hormone which has a major effect on milk production by the mammary glands and is also known as mammotrophin. All basophils produce glycoproteins; some produce TSH and

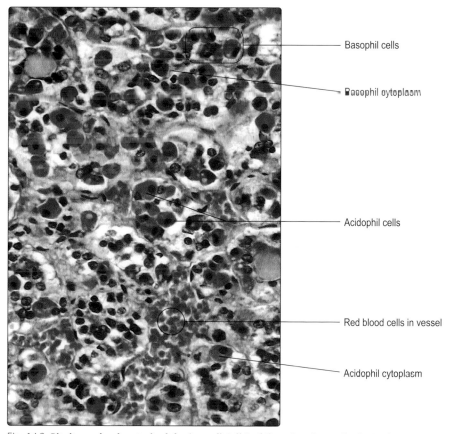

Fig. 14.2 **Pituitary gland, anterior lobe (pars distalis) of the adenohypophysis.** High magnification.

Basophil cells

Basophil cytoplasm

Acidophil cells

Red blood cells in vessel

Acidophil cytoplasm

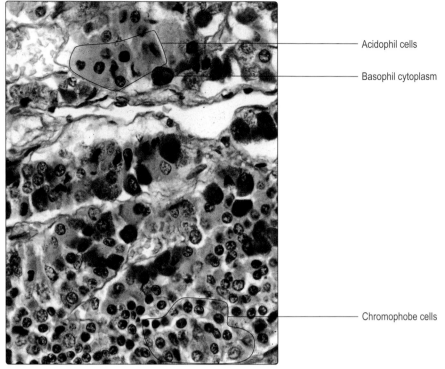

Fig. 14.3 **Pituitary gland, anterior lobe (pars distalis) of the adenohypophysis.**
Glycoproteins in the cytoplasm of basophil cells are stained purplish. The cytoplasm of acidophil cells is stained orangey brown. Some chromophobes have palely stained cytoplasm, others appear to have very little cytoplasm. Special stain. High magnification.

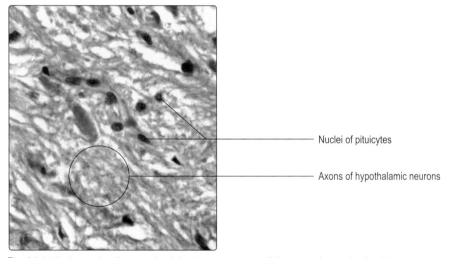

Fig. 14.4 **Pituitary gland, posterior lobe (pars nervosa) of the neurohypophysis.** Pituicytes and axons. High magnification.

others produce adrenocorticotrophic hormone (ACTH), which stimulate, respectively, the thyroid gland and the cells in the cortex of the adrenal glands (see below). Yet other basophils produce two trophic hormones per cell, both categorised as gonadotrophins as they affect endocrine secretion by cells in the gonads (ovaries and testes). The gonadotrophins are follicle-stimulating hormone (FSH) and luteinising hormone (LH). Further details of the function of FSH and LH are described in Chapters 15 and 16.

The pituitary gland is sometimes referred to as the 'conductor of the endocrine orchestra' and this term has also been applied to the hypothalamus. They both have coordinating roles in determining the function of many and varied endocrine-secreting cells in the body. In turn, however, many hormones produced by endocrine cells in endocrine glands and in other organs in the body are able to regulate the secretory activity of cells in the hypothalamus and/or the hypophysis that are stimulating their own levels of hormone production. This type of regulatory mechanism is known as negative feedback (Fig. 14.1).

Neurohypophysis

The neurohypophysis is described in three parts: the median eminence, the infundibulum and the pars nervosa (posterior lobe of the pituitary) (Fig. 14.1).

- *Median eminence.* This part of the hypothalamus contains:
  - neurons that secrete the hypothalamic releasing hormones which regulate the secretory activity of cells in the pars distalis of the pituitary
  - the primary capillary bed of the portal system which carries these hypothalamic hormones to the pars distalis
  - other hormone-producing neuronal cell bodies which have axons that extend along the infundibulum to the pars nervosa.
- *Infundibulum.* This is a continuation of the hypothalamus along the pituitary stalk.
- *Pars nervosa.* This is the region where axons from neurons in the median eminence terminate (Fig. 14.4). Hormones synthesised by these neuronal cell bodies pass along their axons and are stored in granules in swollen axon terminals, known as Herring bodies, before release. These axons are supported by glial cells, called pituicytes. Two hormones are released from the pars nervosa. They are antidiuretic hormone, which acts on the kidneys, and oxytocin, which acts on mammary glands and the uterus. The effects of these hormones are described in Chapters 13 and 16.

Thyroid gland

The thyroid gland lies anterior to the lower part of the larynx and upper trachea. It comprises two lobes that are connected across the mid-line by the isthmus. The majority of the endocrine-secreting cells of the thyroid are arranged as simple (single layered) epithelia surrounding roughly spherical spaces filled with colloid (Fig. 14.5). The colloid is formed by thyroglobulin, an iodinated glycoprotein which is stored as the precursor of active thyroid hormones. These spheres, known as thyroid follicles, vary in size and virtually fill the thyroid gland. Scattered amongst the epithelial cells lining follicles, and in between some follicles, a minor cell population known as parafollicular (C)

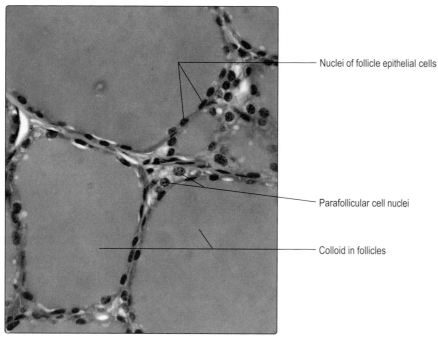

Nuclei of follicle epithelial cells

Parafollicular cell nuclei

Colloid in follicles

Fig. 14.5 **Thyroid gland.** The thyroxine-secreting cells lining these follicles are very flattened and little cytoplasm is apparent. The parafollicular cells have pale staining cytoplasm. High magnification.

cells is present (Fig. 14.5). Parafollicular cells secrete a peptide hormone, calcitonin, which lowers blood calcium levels.

Extracellular storage of hormone precursor molecules in follicles is unique to the thyroid and involves the epithelial cells lining the follicles in numerous complex activities. The appearance of these epithelial cells depends on how active they are. Less active or inactive cells are low, cuboidal or flattened and have few organelles. Active thyroid epithelial cells are columnar and have two main functions; both can occur in the same cell at the same time. They are:

- *Formation and storage of thyroglobulin.* This involves:
  - synthesis of glycoproteins, which are the precursors of thyroglobulin
  - uptake of iodide from blood
  - exocytosis of the glycoproteins into follicles
  - formation of thyroglobulin by the iodination (of tyrosine components) of the glycoproteins as they enter the follicles.
- *Formation and secretion of active thyroid hormone molecules.* This involves:
  - uptake of thyroglobulin from follicles by endocytosis
  - fusion of endocytotic vesicles with lysosomes
  - digestion of thyroglobulin by lysosomes, thus forming active thyroid hormones

- secretion of active thyroid hormones into capillaries.

Thyroxine is the major hormone secreted by thyroid epithelial cells. Thyroxine is derived from iodinated tyrosine molecules in thyroglobulin and is also known tetra-iodothyronine (T4). Thyroxine stimulates metabolism, particularly of carbohydrates and lipids, and promotes growth and development.

Thyroxine levels in blood are controlled by mechanisms involving TrH from the hypothalamus and TSH from the anterior lobe of the pituitary gland (Fig. 14.1). A low level of thyroxine in blood stimulates the secretion of TrH and TSH. The action of TSH on thyroid epithelial cells stimulates the secretion of thyroxine into blood. When the level of thyroxine in blood is too high, negative feedback is activated and thyroxine, acting on the hypothalamus and the hypophysis, suppresses, respectively, the levels of TrH and TSH secreted (Fig. 14.1). The consequence of this feedback is that secretion of thyroxine decreases and blood levels are lowered.

Parafollicular cells in the thyroid are larger than follicular epithelial cells (Fig. 14.5). They secrete the peptide hormone calcitonin directly into capillaries. Calcitonin secretion is stimulated by high levels of calcium in blood and its actions help lower blood calcium. Calcitonin, along with parathyroid hormone (see below), maintains calcium homeostasis. Calcium is essential for many body functions, e.g. the conduction of nerve impulses and contraction of muscle. Regulating the amount of calcium in blood is essential for normal nerve and muscle function.

Parathyroid glands

The parathyroid glands are small paired structures on the posterior surface of the thyroid gland. (There is usually more than one pair.) There are two major parenchymal cell types, chief cells and oxyphil cells (Fig. 14.6). Chief cells are relatively small and make and secrete parathyroid hormone (PTH). Oxyphil cells are larger and stain with dyes such as eosin; their role is not known. In adults, adipocytes appear in the gland (Fig. 14.6).

PTH assists in maintenance of calcium levels in the blood and in body fluids, in conjunction with calcitonin. Low levels of calcium in blood stimulate the secretion of PTH. Calcitonin and PTH have opposite effects and together affect the mineralisation of bone via the activity of osteoclasts (Chapter 9).

Adrenal (suprarenal) glands

The paired adrenal glands are adjacent to the superior surfaces of the kidneys in humans and are known as suprarenal glands. Each gland is composed of an inner medulla surrounded by a much larger outer cortex. A connective tissue capsule surrounds each gland. The cortex and medulla develop from different embryological origins but both secrete hormones. The cortex is derived from embryonic mesoderm and the medulla from neural crest cells. Steroid hormones are produced and secreted by cortical cells, and vasoactive amines by cells in the medulla.

Adrenal cortex

The location of endocrine cells, fenestrated capillaries and reticulin connective tissue in the suprarenal cortex shows three main regions or zonae. They are:

■ *Zona glomerulosa*. This is a narrow region just beneath the capsule formed by roughly spherical clusters of endocrine cells supported by reticulin fibres (Fig. 14.7). Arterioles supply blood to capillaries in this region.

■ *Zona fasciculata*. This is the largest region and it occupies the mid-portion of the cortex. It is characterised by rows of endocrine cells (Figs. 14.7 and 14.8), supported by reticulin fibres, lying alongside straight capillaries extending from capillaries in the zona glomerulosa. The endocrine cells in this zone are known as spongiocytes as their cytoplasm appears vacuolated in routine histological sections (Figs 14.7 and 14.8). The apparently empty vacuoles contained lipids in life, e.g. cholesterol, stored as a precursor for the synthesis of hormones. The lipids were extracted during histological processing.

■ *Zona reticularis*. This is the inner region of the cortex and it surrounds the medulla. The endocrine cells in this region are relatively small (Fig. 14.8) and generally the nucleus and cytoplasm are densely stained. These endocrine cells are distributed irregularly on a reticulin meshwork between capillaries which are continuous with those in the zona fasciculata.

Three groups of steroid hormone, known as corticosteroids, are produced from cholesterol by the endocrine cells in the adrenal cortex. The hormones are not stored in the cells but are synthesised when needed. The three groups of steroid hormone are distinguished by their functions.

■ *Mineralocorticoids*. The molecules in this group regulate water and salt concentration via actions on the distal convoluted tubules of the kidney (Chapter 13). The major mineralocorticoid hormone is aldosterone and it is produced mainly by cells in the zona glomerulosa.

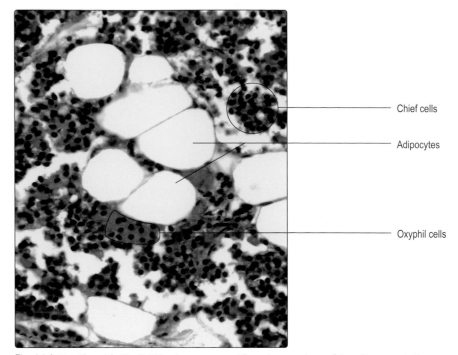

Fig. 14.6 **Parathyroid.** The lipid has been extracted from the cytoplasm of the adipocytes during processing. High magnification.

— Chief cells
— Adipocytes
— Oxyphil cells

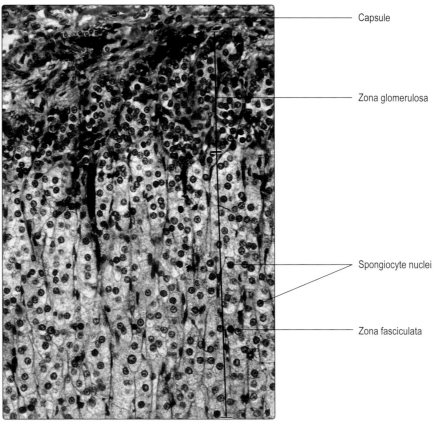

Fig. 14.7 **Adrenal gland, zona glomerulosa and zona fasciculata of the cortex.** Connective tissue is stained blue. Special stain. Medium magnification.

— Capsule
— Zona glomerulosa
— Spongiocyte nuclei
— Zona fasciculata

- *Glucocorticoids*. This group of hormones is mainly produced by cells in the zona fasciculata. One of the principal glucocorticoids is cortisol. Glucocorticoid hormones affect many target cells and are involved in regulating the metabolism of carbohydrates, fats and proteins. They are also able to suppress immune responses.
- *Sex hormones*. These steroids are produced mainly by cells in the zona reticularis. Most of the molecules are male sex hormones of low activity.

The secretion of hormones by the adrenal cortex is under the regulatory control of ACTH from the anterior lobe of the pituitary gland. In turn, ACTH secretion is controlled by a releasing hormone (corticotrophin rH) from the hypothalamus. High levels of cortico-steroids in blood suppress secretion of corticotrophin rH and ACTH. In addition, mineralocorticoid levels are affected by the intake of various mineral salts.

Adrenal medulla

The medulla of the adrenal gland is surrounded by the zona reticularis of the cortex. Medullary endocrine cells are modified postganglionic sympathetic neurons; they do not have axons. In general, medullary cells are large and in clusters or cords (Fig. 14.8) near capillaries and are supported by reticulin fibres. The medulla receives blood from arterioles and from capillaries extending in from the zona reticularis. All blood from the cortex drains into veins in the medulla (Fig. 14.8). There are two principal hormones synthesised by the endocrine cells in the medulla, adrenaline and noradrenaline; both are vasoactive amines. Each hormone is stored in small quantities in cytoplasmic granules. Release of hormones is stimulated by preganglionic nerves acting on the endocrine cells in the medulla. Under stressful conditions, much larger amounts of medullary hormones may be released.

Pancreas

The pancreas is a flattish organ in the abdominal cavity. The bulk of the pancreas is formed by exocrine cells and their secretions enter the gastrointestinal tract at the duodenum via the pancreatic duct (Chapter 12). The pancreas also contains endocrine cells in small clusters known as islets of Langerhans (Fig. 14.9). There are about a million islets scattered throughout the pancreas.

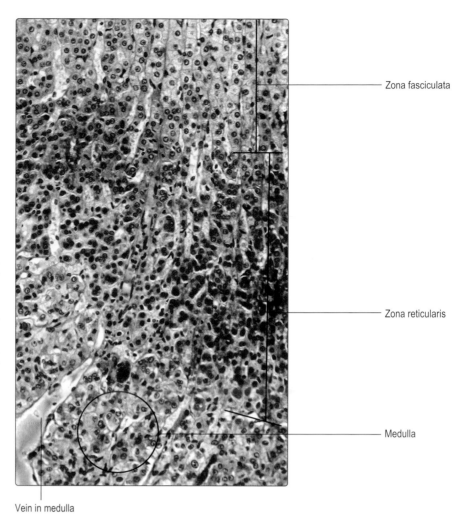

Zona fasciculata
Zona reticularis
Medulla
Vein in medulla

Fig. 14.8 **Adrenal gland, zona fasciculata, zona reticularis of the cortex and medulla.** Connective tissue is stained blue. Special stain. Medium magnification.

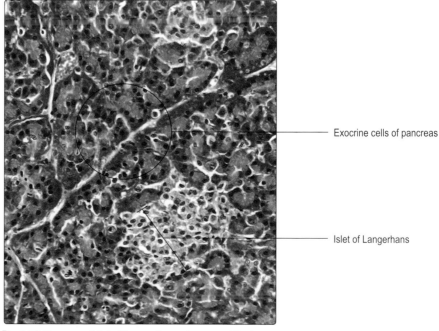

Exocrine cells of pancreas
Islet of Langerhans

Fig. 14.9 **Pancreas, islet of Langerhans.** Low magnification.

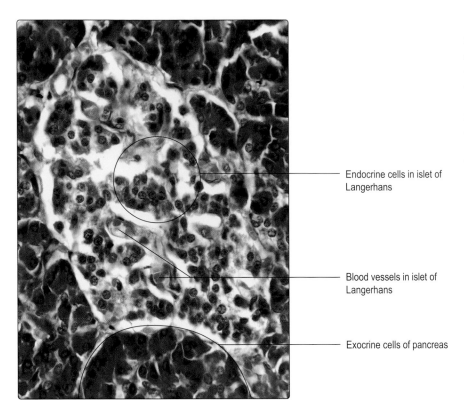

Endocrine cells in islet of Langerhans

Blood vessels in islet of Langerhans

Exocrine cells of pancreas

Fig. 14.10 **Pancreas, islet of Langerhans.** High magnification.

Islets of Langerhans generally are seen in histological sections as pale staining areas in comparison with surrounding exocrine cells (Figs 14.9 and 14.10). The endocrine cells lie close to capillaries (Fig. 14.10) and several types have been identified. All the hormones produced are involved in regulating carbohydrate metabolism and other aspects of the functions of the digestive system. Immunohistochemical techniques have shown several cell types in each islet, each type secreting a different hormone. Most of the cells secrete insulin and are known as beta cells. Insulin, a polypeptide, reduces blood glucose levels. The next most populous cell type, alpha cells, secretes another polypeptide, glucagon, which elevates blood glucose levels. Other minority cell populations are involved in regulating gastrointestinal tract function.

The factors affecting endocrine secretion by the pancreas are numerous. One of the major factors affecting insulin secretion is the level of glucose in blood. In addition, sympathetic nerves inhibit insulin secretion and, conversely, parasympathetic nerves increase insulin secretion.

Pineal gland

The pineal gland is closely associated with the brain. Despite this proximity, and in contrast to the pituitary gland, there are no nerves which directly connect the pineal gland and the brain. The pineal gland responds to changes in light levels. It is concerned with the regulation of circadian rhythm, and is influenced by hormones from the gonads. The main cell types are pinealocytes and interstitial cells. Pinealocytes produce melatonin in the absence of light. The interstitial cells may be similar to glial cells.

Clinical note

All endocrine glands may secrete abnormally high, or low, levels of hormones. There are numerous causes. Malignant changes in endocrine cells can result in abnormal levels of hormone production. In other instances, abnormal levels of a particular pituitary trophic hormone, e.g. TSH, may be caused by inadequate levels of hormone production by other cells, e.g. inadequate levels of TrH from the hypothalamus. In some cases, an abnormal (auto)antibody may develop which binds to a particular circulating hormone and affects the function of that hormone. Some autoantibodies affect the thyroid gland and result in hypothyroidism manifest as Hashimoto's disease.

Summary

The endocrine system

Hypothalamus and hypophysis (pituitary gland)

- The hypothalamus is the part of the brain connected by a (pituitary) stalk to the hypophysis.
- The hypophysis has a glandular portion (adenohypophysis) and neural portion (neurohypophysis).
- Some hypothalamic hormones (peptides) affect the function of the adenohypophysis:
  - neurons in the hypothalamus secrete releasing hormones into capillaries in the hypothalamus which pass (in a portal circulation) along the stalk and stimulate the release of hormones from cells in the adenohypophysis
- Other neurons in the hypothalamus produce hormones (peptides) which pass via their axons (along the stalk) to the neurohypophysis.
- Feedback signals from the levels of hormones in blood affect the secretion of most hypothalamic and hypophyseal hormones.

Adenohypophysis

- Chromophil and chromophobe cells are present:
  - acidophil cells secrete growth hormone or prolactin (proteins)
  - basophil cells secrete thyroid-stimulating hormone or adrenocorticotrophic hormone or follicle-stimulating hormone and luteinising hormone (glycoproteins).
- Chromophobe function is not understood

Neurohypophysis

- Pituicytes support axons from neurons with cell bodies in the hypothalamus.
- Hypothalamic hormones antidiuretic hormone (ADH) and oxytocin are stored in the ends of the axons (as Herring bodies):
  - ADH affects kidney tubules and decreases the amount of water excreted
  - oxytocin stimulates lactation and contraction of uterine smooth muscle.

Thyroid

- A simple epithelium synthesises, secretes and stores thyroglobulin (an iodinated protein) as colloid in spherical follicles.
- These epithelial cells also endocytose the thyroglobulin, convert it into active thyroid hormones (e.g. thyroxine) and secrete them into blood vessels:
  - thyroid hormones stimulate metabolism.
- Parafollicular cells secrete the peptide hormone calcitonin directly into blood when blood calcium levels are high. Calcitonin lowers calcium levels in blood.

Parathyroid glands

- Chief cells secrete parathyroid hormone when blood calcium is low, which raises calcium levels via its stimulation of the activity of osteoclasts. Oxyphil and adipose cells are also present.

Adrenal glands

- Adrenal cortex synthesises, secretes steroids:
  - zona glomerulosa cells secrete mineralocorticoids which affect salt balance
  - zona fasciculata cells (spongiocytes) secrete glucocorticoids which regulate metabolism and are immunosuppressive
  - zona reticularis cells secrete, male sex hormones of low activity.
- Adrenal medulla secretes vasoactive amines:
  - cells are modified sympathetic neurons which secrete adrenaline or noradrenaline involved in responses (fright, fight and flight) to stress.

Pancreas

- Islets of Langerhans cells secrete hormones (peptides) which affect carbohydrate metabolism. Insulin is secreted by beta cells and it reduces blood glucose levels. Glucagon is secreted by alpha cells and it raises blood glucose levels.

Pineal gland

- Responds to light, secretes melatonin and helps regulate circadian rhythm.

Chapter 15
The male reproductive system

The male reproductive system comprises paired testes, associated glands, ducts and the penis (Fig. 15.1). The testes are the male gonads and are the site of production of spermatozoa (the male gametes). Each spermatozoon (in humans) has 23 chromosomes containing the haploid amount of DNA. Additionally, testes produce and secrete a group of steroid hormones, the male sex hormones (androgens), of which testosterone is the main type. The glands that are associated with the male reproductive system are the paired seminal vesicles, the prostate and paired bulbourethral glands. All these glands contribute fluid secretions which support spermatozoa and form semen. The ducts form the reproductive tract and transport spermatozoa and secretions from the testes and glands to the urethra. The urethra is shared by the reproductive and urinary systems and it passes from the bladder through the prostate and penis and opens at a meatus at the glans penis. The urethra transports urine from the urinary bladder as it is emptied at micturition. The penis is also

the organ of copulation able to deliver spermatozoa, in semen, into the vagina of the female reproductive tract.

Testes

Each testis is an organ suspended within a pouch of skin known as the scrotum. The testes thus lie outside the abdominal cavity and this ensures that spermatogenesis (the formation of spermatozoa) occurs at a temperature slightly below body temperature, a requirement for successful gamete production. Each testis is surrounded by a tough connective tissue covering known as the tunica albuginea. Connective tissue septa from the tunica albuginea penetrate into the substance of each testis and divide it into lobules. One septum forms a wedge which penetrates the posterior surface of each testis.

Seminiferous tubules
Located within the lobules of each testis are coiled seminiferous tubules which are the sites of spermatogenesis. Sem-

iniferous tubules are lined by several layers of epithelial cells forming a germinal (seminiferous) epithelium (Fig. 15.2). There are two types of cell in the germinal epithelium of adults: spermatogenic cells, which are in layers, and Sertoli cells, which form a single layer and are supportive of the spermatogenic cells (see below). The germinal epithelium lies on a basement membrane and is surrounded by a thin layer of loose connective tissue. This connective tissue supports blood vessels (Fig. 15.2), lymph capillaries, nerves and Leydig (interstitial) cells (Fig. 15.3) which secrete androgens (see below). Myoid cells (Fig. 15.4) are closely adjacent to seminiferous tubules and are capable of contraction, thus helping to move the spermatozoa along tubules and away from where they develop.

After puberty, spermatogenesis begins as spermatogenic cells undergo meiosis and differentiation in a cycle of events that result in the production of spermatozoa, a process which takes about 65 days in humans. The stages of spermatogenesis take different lengths of time

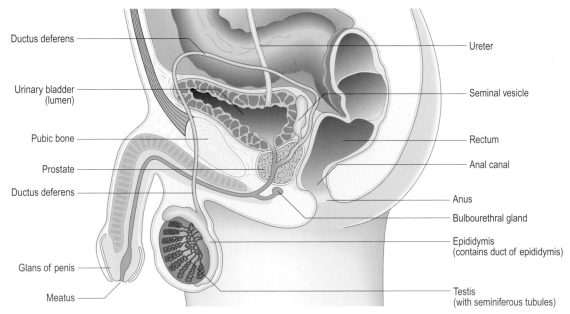

Fig. 15.1 **The component parts of the male reproductive system.**

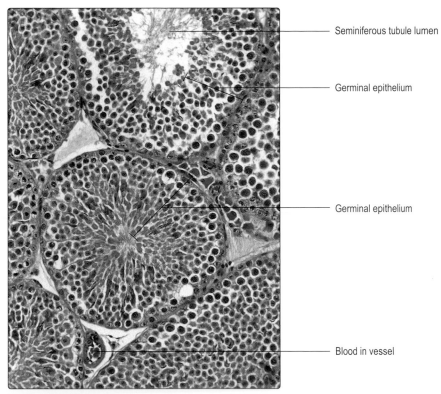

Fig. 15.2 **Testis. Seminiferous tubules.** One tubule appears circular as it is sectioned across its length. Medium magnification.

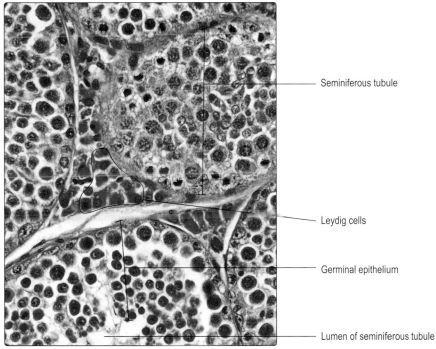

Fig. 15.3 **Testis. Seminiferous tubules and Leydig (interstitial) cells.** High magnification.

to complete and, as a result, not all the stages are present in the layers of cells in any one region of the germinal epithelium. The appearance of seminiferous tubules depends on the stages the spermatogenic cells have reached in forming spermatozoa and on the angle at which they are sectioned (Figs 15.2 and 15.5).

Spermatogenic cells

The formation of spermatozoa (spermatogenesis) may be divided into three stages: mitosis, meiosis and spermiogenesis. These stages begin at about puberty and continue throughout life.

■ *Mitosis.* In this stage, stem cells (spermatogonia) at the base of the germinal epithelium undergo regular cycles of mitosis and produce new diploid cells, i.e. cells containing the normal number of chromosomes (46 in humans, comprising 22 homologous pairs and two sex chromosomes). Some of the new cells formed by mitosis remain in the basal layer as spermatogonia, others move towards the lumen and enter meiosis.

■ *Meiosis.* At the start of this phase the cells begin to enlarge and are known as primary spermatocytes. They undergo an S phase when they replicate the DNA in their chromosomes prior to cell division (Chapter 2). They then enter the prophase of the first division in meiosis (Fig. 15.6), a process which lasts about 20 days. During this time, chromosomes begin to coil and condense (and stain densely) and homologous pairs of chromosomes move close together and exchange lengths of DNA. This exchange introduces genetic variation to the gametes produced.

The first meiotic division of meiosis (also known as the reduction division) continues into metaphase. Each pair of homologous chromosomes in each primary spermatocyte line up together on the same part of the equator of the spindle of the metaphase plate, prior to cell division. (This contrasts with mitosis, where each chromosome attaches to a different part of the equator of the spindle.) At this stage, the chromosomes are at their most condensed and densely stained and are readily identified in histological sections (Fig. 15.7). The paired chromosomes then move away from each other in anaphase and telophase. The result of this reduction division is the production of two secondary spermatocytes each with only half the original number of chromosomes (i.e. 23 in humans). (This reduction division introduces further genetic variation to the new cells as maternally and paternally derived chromosomes in the homologous pairs are randomly arranged on the spindle, and therefore randomly distributed between the two offspring cells.)

The second meiotic division, known as the mitotic division of meiosis, occurs rapidly as chromosomes in secondary spermatocytes line up as individuals

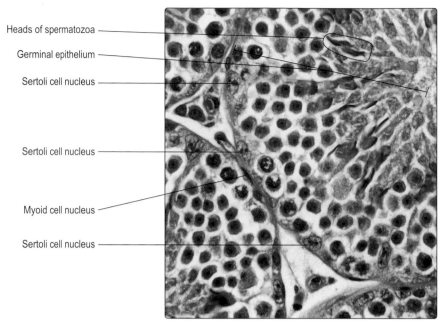

Heads of spermatozoa

Germinal epithelium

Sertoli cell nucleus

Sertoli cell nucleus

Myoid cell nucleus

Sertoli cell nucleus

Fig. 15.4 **Testis. Seminiferous tubules, Sertoli cells and myoid cells.** Sertoli cell nuclei are pale staining and nucleoli are present. Myoid cells are identified by their long thin nuclei lying adjacent to the base of the germinal epithelium. High magnification.

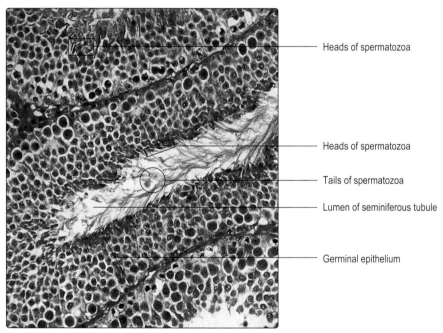

Heads of spermatozoa

Heads of spermatozoa

Tails of spermatozoa

Lumen of seminiferous tubule

Germinal epithelium

Fig. 15.5 **Testis. Seminiferous tubules.** The lumen of one seminiferous tubule is sectioned along its length. The similarity of the cells in the layers of the germinal epithelium around the tubule reflect their synchronisation in the stages of forming spermatozoa. At this magnification heads of spermatozoa appear as very small blue dots, adjacent to the lumen, but it is not possible to see their individual tails. Medium magnification.

(as they do in mitosis) on the metaphase spindle of this division. The chromosomes then split (along their length) and separate into two new cells, known as spermatids. As this cell division is rapid, few cells in any one histological section are in this phase. Each resulting spermatid has 23 chromosomes with the haploid amount of DNA. This is half the number of chromosomes and half the DNA in the stem cells (spermatogonia), and of most other cells in the body.

Separation of cytoplasm during meiosis is incomplete and spermatids derived from one spermatogonium are partially joined together. This is thought to aid synchrony of their progression through the next stage (spermiogenesis). Groups of newly formed, related spermatids appear as clusters of small, spherical cells near the luminal surface of seminiferous tubules (Fig. 15.6).

- *Spermiogenesis.* During this stage, spermatids differentiate and each forms one spermatozoon. Approximately 200 million spermatozoa are produced daily by the testes in humans. During spermiogenesis the spherical spermatids change in form and shed cytoplasm as they become highly differentiated spermatozoa characterised by a head, middle region and tail (Fig. 15.8). As spermatozoa develop, the head regions remain in the epithelium but the tail regions extend into the lumen of the seminiferous tubule (Fig. 15.5). Eventually, spermatozoa pass into the lumen and fluid secreted by Sertoli cells (see below) aids their transport away from the seminiferous tubules.

The head of each spermatozoon contains the nucleus in which the DNA in the chromosomes is condensed and stains densely with bases such as haematoxylin (Figs 15.4, 15.5 and 15.6). At one end of the nucleus of a developing spermatozoon a head 'cap' develops known as the acrosome (Fig. 15.8). The contents of the acrosome include hydrolytic enzymes that take part in the acrosome reaction, which is the process by which the head of a spermatozoon penetrates the cells and structures surrounding the oocyte prior to fertilisation (Chapter 16). The middle region of a spermatozoon is mainly occupied by mitochondria which provide energy for the movement of the tail (flagellum) (Fig. 15.8). The tail has the 9 + 2 arrangement of microtubules characteristic of cilia (Chapter 2), and these provide the motive force which allows spermatozoa to swim. However, spermatozoa become self-propelled only after they have left the testes and are fully matured, when they are then able to undertake unidirectional travel at about 3 mm/minute.

Sertoli cells

Sertoli cells are tall and columnar, and extend from the base of the germinal epithelium to the lumen of the seminiferous tubule (Fig. 15.10). The nucleus of Sertoli cells may appear oval or triangular and most display a prominent

Fig. 15.6 **Testis. Seminiferous tubules, primary spermatocytes and spermatids.** Primary spermatocytes in prophase of the first meiotic (reduction) division are distinguished by their large size and speckled, clumped chromatin. High magnification.

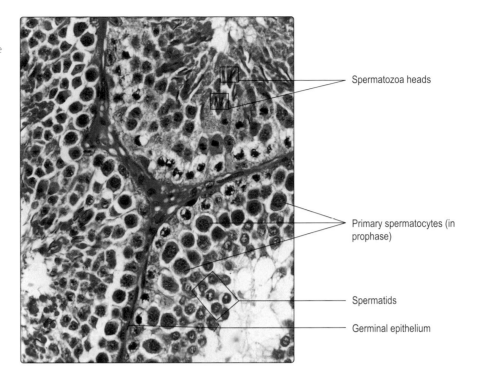

— Spermatozoa heads

— Primary spermatocytes (in prophase)

— Spermatids

— Germinal epithelium

Fig. 15.7 **Testis. Seminiferous tubules, primary spermatocytes undergoing cell division.** Note the difference in the types of cell in the epithelium on opposite sides of the lumen; dividing cells are only in one region. Clusters of cells are in synchrony but at different stages of forming spermatozoa in different parts of the tubule. High magnification.

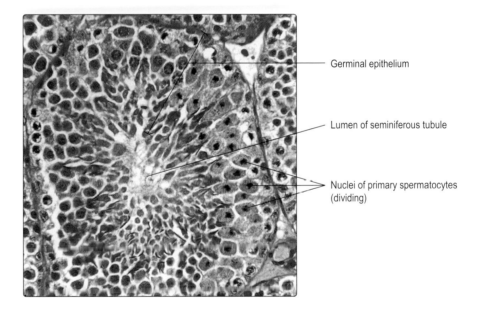

— Germinal epithelium

— Lumen of seminiferous tubule

— Nuclei of primary spermatocytes (dividing)

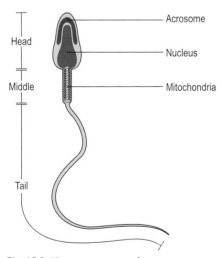

— Acrosome

— Nucleus

— Mitochondria

Head

Middle

Tail

Fig. 15.8 **The components of a spermatozoon.**

nucleolus and palely stained chromatin, reflecting their high levels of synthetic activity (Figs 15.4 and 15.9). Developing spermatogenic cells are enfolded in the lateral cell membranes of Sertoli cells and as a result detail of Sertoli cell structure is difficult to distinguish in routine histological sections. Adjacent Sertoli cells are joined to each other near to the basement membrane by tight junctions (Fig. 15.10). This arrangement separates spermatogonia into a basal compartment of the germinal epithelium and the developing spermatogenic cells (from primary spermatocytes to spermatozoa) into an adluminal compartment. The barrier formed between the two compartments is known as the blood–testis barrier and it ensures that large molecules, e.g. antibodies or microorganisms in blood, do not readily pass to developing spermatozoa.

Sertoli cells are also important in nourishing developing spermatogenic cells and they phagocytose cytoplasmic fragments released from spermatozoa as they develop. An important component in the secretions from Sertoli cells is an androgen-binding protein. This binds testosterone and helps to ensure levels in the seminiferous tubules are higher than in the circulation and at a level adequate for the development of spermatozoa. In addition, fluid secreted

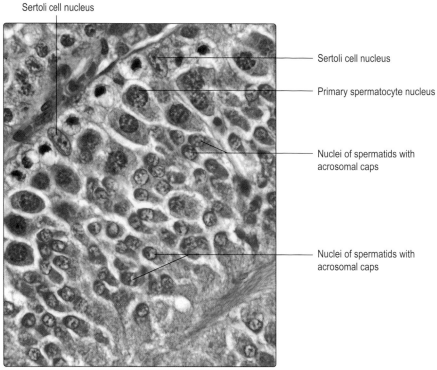

Sertoli cell nucleus

- Sertoli cell nucleus
- Primary spermatocyte nucleus
- Nuclei of spermatids with acrosomal caps
- Nuclei of spermatids with acrosomal caps

Fig. 15.9 **Testis. Seminiferous tubule with Sertoli cells and spermatids developing acrosomes.** High magnification.

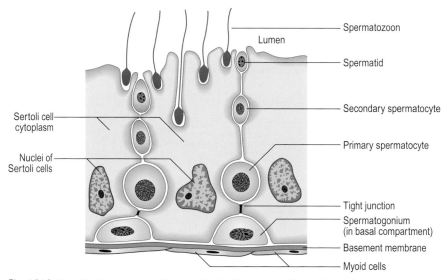

- Spermatozoon
Lumen
- Spermatid
- Secondary spermatocyte
- Primary spermatocyte

Sertoli cell cytoplasm

Nuclei of Sertoli cells

- Tight junction
- Spermatogonium (in basal compartment)
- Basement membrane
- Myoid cells

Fig. 15.10 **Sertoli cells in a seminiferous tubule.** The relationship of adjacent Sertoli cells is shown forming a basal compartment containing spermatogonia and an adluminal compartment containing developing spermatozoa closely associated with the Sertoli cells.

Clinical note

Infertility There are numerous causes of infertility. Low numbers of spermatozoa in an ejaculate is one reason why infertility occurs. Malnutrition and alcoholism are factors which also affect fertility.

Immotile cilia syndrome is a state which affects all the ciliated cells in the body as well as the flagellum of each spermatozoon. The inability of spermatozoa to move and reach an oocyte in the uterine tube will affect fertility. A person with immotile cilia is also likely to suffer from frequent respiratory tract infections as inhaled microorganisms are not swept along the mucus escalator and away from the lungs.

by Sertoli cells helps to move spermatozoa away from the testis as at this stage the spermatozoa are not able to propel themselves.

Variations in germinal epithelium
Various groupings of cells at the same stages of spermatogenesis occur in different regions of the seminiferous tubules. For example, in some regions (Fig. 15.5) the condensed heads of spermatozoa before they are released into the lumen are apparent, whereas in other regions none of the developing spermatids has condensed chromatin (Fig. 15.9). These groupings of similar cells developing in synchrony occur as lengths (Fig. 15.5) or as patches of the epithelium (Fig. 15.7) in humans. This variation ensures that mature spermatozoa are continuously produced and always available for release at ejaculation.

Leydig (interstitial) cells
Leydig cells are endocrine cells in the loose connective tissue around seminiferous tubules (Fig. 15.3) and they secrete mainly testosterone. The Leydig cells are stimulated to produce and secrete testosterone by luteinising hormone secreted by cells in the anterior pituitary gland (Chapter 14). Testosterone enters the circulation and stimulates secondary sexual characteristics including skeletal muscle development and the pattern of hair growth. However, circulating levels of testosterone are insufficient to maintain spermatogenesis. Testosterone levels in the testis are kept high enough to stimulate spermatogenesis as the androgen-binding protein secreted by Sertoli cells binds testosterone in the testis. Another hormone from anterior pituitary cells, follicle-stimulating hormone, stimulates Sertoli cells to secrete the androgen-binding protein.

Ducts draining seminiferous tubules
Most seminiferous tubules are coiled loops which have straight regions (tubuli recti) at each end through which fluid and spermatozoa leave. The tubuli recti drain into a meshwork of spaces, lined by cubodial epithelium, known as the rete testis. The rete is embedded in the wedge of connective tissue which extends into each testis from the tunica albuginea. The contents of the rete testis drain into 12 to 15 ductuli efferentes, which in turn drain into a single duct in the epididymis.

Ducts draining each testis (Fig. 15.1)

Ductus epididymis

Each ductus epididymis is a highly convoluted tubule surrounded by a thin layer of smooth muscle cells. Each is tightly packed in an epididymis by connective tissue and attached to the posterior surface of a testis. At the superior pole of each testis is the head of the epididymis where ductuli efferentes drain fluid and spermatozoa from each testis into the duct of the epididymis. From the lower pole of each testis (the tail of the epididymis) the duct of the epididymis continues as the ductus (vas) deferens (see below).

The epithelium lining the ductus epididymis is pseudostratified and composed of basal and columnar epithelial (principal) cells (Fig. 15.11). The basal cells are stem cells from which the columnar cells are derived. Large cytoplasmic processes, known as stereocilia, extend from the surface of the columnar cells. Stereocilia do not have the structure or function of cilia; instead, they function as microvilli and resorb fluid and remnants of cytoplasm from developing spermatozoa. This fluid resorption and contraction of smooth muscle around the ductus epididymis (Fig. 15.11) facilitate the movement of spermatozoa away from the testis and towards the ductus deferens.

Ductus deferens

Each ductus deferens is a thick muscular tube that conducts fluid and spermatozoa at ejaculation from a ductus epididymis into an ejaculatory duct in the prostate. At the ejaculatory duct, secretions from a seminal vesicle and the prostate gland are added to the ejaculate and the combined contents (seminal fluid) enter the urethra, where it passes through the prostate.

Each ductus deferens is lined by a pseudostratified columnar epithelium similar to that of the epididymis. There are three thick layers of smooth muscle surrounding the ductus deferens arranged as inner and outer longitudinal layers and a middle circular layer (Fig. 15.12). Contraction of this relatively large amount of smooth muscle is initiated and coordinated by sympathetic nerves and it ensures that strong contractions propel the seminal fluid along the ductus deferens and on through the urethra at ejaculation.

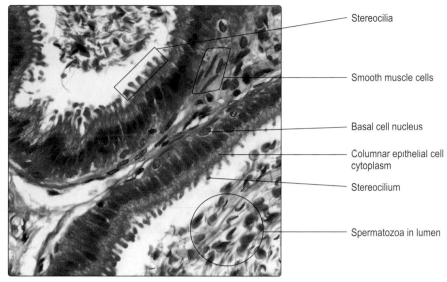

Fig. 15.11 **Ductus epididymis.** High magnification.

Stereocilia
Smooth muscle cells
Basal cell nucleus
Columnar epithelial cell cytoplasm
Stereocilium
Spermatozoa in lumen

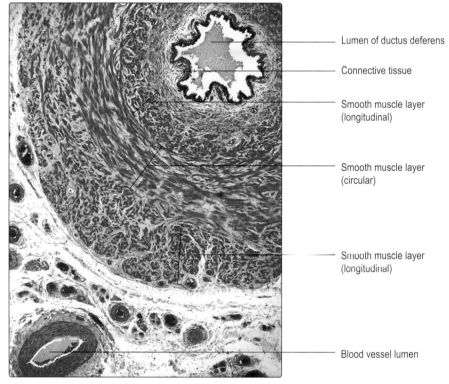

Fig. 15.12 **Ductus deferens.** Very low magnification.

Lumen of ductus deferens
Connective tissue
Smooth muscle layer (longitudinal)
Smooth muscle layer (circular)
Smooth muscle layer (longitudinal)
Blood vessel lumen

Glands of the male reproductive system

Prostate

The prostate is a glandular structure that lies beneath the urinary bladder and surrounds part of the urethra. It is a compound tubuloalveolar gland (Chapter 3) whose epithelium is supported by a fibroelastic stroma which contains numerous irregularly arranged smooth muscle cells (Fig. 15.13). The whole organ is surrounded by a connective tissue capsule. The gland is described in three zones (outer, middle and inner

zones) (Fig. 15.14). The largest zone is the outer zone, and the inner is the smallest. The secretions drain either directly or via short or longer ducts into the urethra.

The prostatic epithelium is stimulated to secrete by testosterone. It varies in appearance between being a pseudostratified columnar epithelium (Fig. 15.13) when stimulated and a low, simple cuboidal epithelium when testosterone levels are low. The lumina of prostatic glands store the secretions which are emptied into the urethra at ejaculation. The propulsive force that

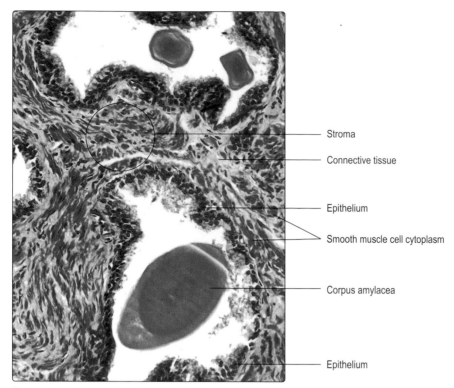

Fig. 15.13 **Prostate gland.** The muscle cells within the stroma stain more intensely pink than the connective tissue cells and fibres. Low magnification.

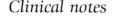

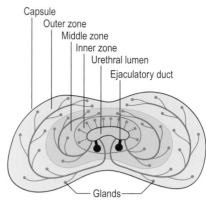

Fig. 15.14 **A transverse section through the prostate and urethra.**

moves the secretions at ejaculation is due to contraction of smooth muscle cells (Fig. 15.13) in the prostatic stroma (under the control of sympathetic nerves). Prostatic secretions contain citric acid, which may provide an energy source for spermatozoa, and various proteins including a form of acid phosphatase unique to the prostate. With age, concretions (corpora amylacea) composed of calcified glycoproteins may be present in the lumina of prostatic glands (Fig. 15.13) but they are of unknown significance.

Seminal vesicles

Paired seminal vesicles are located on the posterior surface of the urinary bladder. Each contains a highly coiled tube which drains into an ejaculatory duct where, at ejaculation, it is added to fluid from a ductus deferens. (Seminal vesicles in humans do not store spermatozoa.)

Each tube within a seminal vesicle is lined by a highly folded epithelium which may appear as a pseudostratified columnar epithelium or simple, low cuboidal epithelium. The appearance and function of the epithelium is affected by the amount of circulating male sex hormones. The epithelial-lined tube in each seminal vesicle is supported by fibroelastic connective tissue. Smooth muscle, arranged as an inner circular and outer longitudinal layer, surrounds the coiled tube and on the exterior of the seminal vesicles there is a layer of loose fibroelastic tissue.

Contraction of the smooth muscle in seminal vesicles, stimulated by sympathetic nerves, propels their secretions into the ejaculate. The secretions from the seminal vesicles are watery and contain fructose, which acts as an essential energy source for spermatozoa. They also contain a lipochrome pigment which imparts a yellowish colour to semen.

Bulbourethral glands

The bulbourethral glands are paired glands that lie at the base of the penis and drain directly into the urethra. They secrete a small volume of mucoid material that precedes the ejaculation of semen and acts as a lubricant along the urethra; it may also assist with lubrication of the vagina during sexual intercourse.

Urethra

In males, the urethra shares urinary and reproductive functions and is longer than the urethra in females, in whom its sole function is to drain urine from the bladder. The urethra in males is described as having three regions: the prostatic, membranous and penile (spongy) urethra. The initial portion,

---

Clinical notes

Benign prostatic hypertrophy This condition afflicts 30–40% of men over the age of 50 years, and more than 95% of men over the age of 80 years. As it is the inner zone of the gland that is affected, any enlargement can readily put pressure on the urethra and affect the ability to pass urine.

Prostate cancer Cancer of the prostate affects about 30% of males over the age of 75 years, and in older men it is almost always present. However, in older men it is usually a very slow growing form of cancer and the individuals usually die from some other disease. In cancer of the prostate, it is usually the outer zone that is affected and, in its most aggressive form, it may spread via the bloodstream before any swelling compresses the urethra and inhibits micturition.

A diagnostic test used to indicate an increased risk of prostatic cancer is a blood test to measure the levels of circulating prostate-specific antigen (PSA). This glycoprotein is secreted by prostatic epithelial cells into the lumina of the glands and normally does not circulate in blood. If prostatic epithelial cells have spread beyond their basement membrane their secretions may circulate in blood. However, PSA may also be raised in patients with benign prostatic hypertrophy, so its usefulness as a diagnostic test is limited.

draining the urinary bladder, is the prostatic urethra. It is lined by transitional epithelium and is surrounded by the prostate. At ejaculation, the prostatic urethra drains secretions from the prostate and the ejaculatory ducts (carrying secretions from seminal vesicles, spermatozoa and fluid from the testes). The membranous part of the urethra is short and connects the prostatic urethra to the penile urethra. It is lined by stratified or pseudostratified columnar epithelium. The penile urethra is the longest region of the urethra. It is also lined by stratified or pseudostratified columnar epithelium (Fig. 15.15) and in places it has deep folds (Fig. 15.16). Near the meatus at the end of the penis the urethral epithelium changes and becomes a stratified non-keratinising squamous epithelium. The lamina propria supporting the epithelium in all regions of the urethra is composed of loose fibroelastic connective tissue.

Penis

The penis consists of three cylinders (corpora) of erectile tissue, each surrounded by a dense fibrous connective tissue sheath (the tunica albuginea) and enclosed by thin skin. One cylinder, the corpus spongiosum, surrounds the penile urethra (Fig. 15.15), and the other two (corpora cavernosa) lie dorsally. The erectile tissue of the corpora consists mainly of interconnecting venous spaces (Fig. 15.17) which are virtually empty when the penis is in its flaccid state.

The penis has a rich blood supply that flows in helicine arteries (Figs 15.15 and 15.17), which are spiral in form in the flaccid state. Most blood, in the flaccid state, flows directly via arteriovenous shunts linking arterioles (supplied by the helicine arteries) directly to deep venules and veins draining the penis. However, some arterial blood perfuses capillaries and thus supplies the penis with oxygen and nutrients. During an erection, the arteriovenous shunts are closed and arterial blood is diverted and fills and swells the venous spaces (Fig. 15.17) in all the corpora. As a result, venous return from the penis is restricted, the penis increases in volume, it lengthens, and the helicine arteries extend. The arrangement of the connective tissue around the corpora (Figs 15.15 and 15.17) ensures that the penis extends as a column. Parasympathetic nerves supplying smooth muscle around arterioles in the penis act as vasodilators and are responsible for the

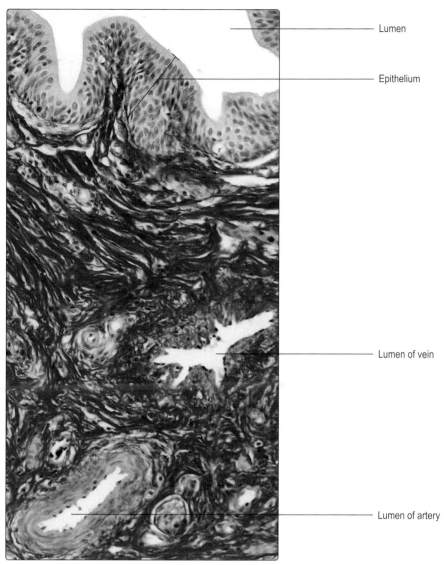

Fig. 15.15 **Penile urethra, corpus spongiosum.** Connective tissue is stained red. Special stain. Medium magnification.

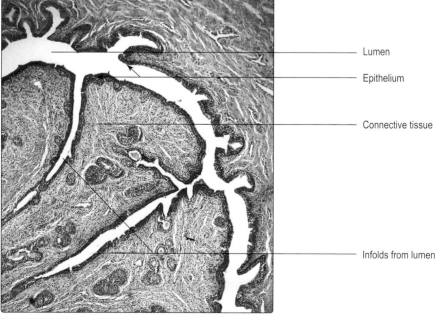

Fig. 15.16 **Penile urethra.** Very low magnification.

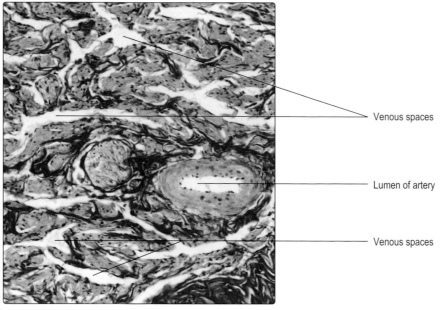

Venous spaces

Lumen of artery

Venous spaces

Fig. 15.17 **Penile urethra, corpus cavernosus.** Connective tissue is stained red. Special stain. Medium magnification.

haemodynamic changes producing an erect penis.

Ejaculation is under the control of sympathetic nerves. They stimulate contraction of smooth muscle cells in the ductus deferens (and other ducts), in the prostate gland and in seminal vesicles. The pressure exerted on the urethra by the engorged corpus spongiosum is less than that in the corpora cavernosa. It is normally sufficient to prevent micturition, but not the powerful propulsion of semen at ejaculation. After ejaculation, sympathetic stimulation ceases and smooth muscle contraction ceases. Parasympathetic stimulation also ceases and this opens the arteriovenous shunts and the flaccid state of the penis is restored.

Summary

The male reproductive system
- This consists of paired testes, ducts, associated glands and the penis.

Testes
- Testes contain coiled seminiferous tubules lined by a stratified germinal epithelium (which produces spermatozoa), Sertoli cells (which support the developing spermatozoa) and Leydig (interstitial) cells (between the tubules) which produce testosterone under the influence of luteinising hormone from the anterior pituitary.

Spermatogenesis
- This is the series of stages involved in producing spermatozoa: it begins at puberty and continues for life.
- Spermatogenesis involves mitosis of stem cells (spermatogonia), meiotic division of spermatocytes and spermiogenesis:
  - some cells produced by mitosis of spermatogonia enter meiosis and become primary spermatocytes; others remain as stem cells
  - primary spermatocytes replicate the DNA of their chromosomes prior to meiotic division
  - in the first division (reduction) of meiosis, a primary spermatocyte divides into two secondary spermatocytes, each with half the original number of chromosomes
  - in the second division (mitotic) of meiosis, each secondary spermatocyte divides into two spermatids, each with half the amount of DNA (and half the original number of chromosomes)
  - spermatids differentiate into spermatozoa (the process of spermiogenesis):
    - spermatozoa each have a head, neck and tail (the tail beats and provides unidirectional propulsion).

Ducts
- Ducts drain spermatozoa and fluid secreted by Sertoli cells from seminiferous tubules.
- Immotile spermatozoa pass from each testis into a ductus epididymis as fluid is absorbed by epithelial cells lining these ducts.
- At ejaculation, spermatozoa pass rapidly from each ductus epididymis into and along a ductus deferens, propelled by the peristaltic contraction of the thick muscle layers surrounding each ductus deferens.

Associated glands
- These add secretions to the ejaculate which provide nutrients for spermatozoa:
  - the prostate gland has smooth muscle in the stroma which contracts and expels the secretions from the epithelial cells
  - the paired seminal vesicles each contain a coiled tubule lined with epithelial cells and surrounded by smooth muscle.

Penis
- The penis comprises three corpora of erectile tissue, each surrounded by a dense fibrous connective tissue sheath and enclosed by thin skin. One cylinder, the corpus spongiosus, surrounds the penile urethra.
  - increased blood flow into the blood vessels in erectile tissue, particularly in the paired corpora cavernosus, produces an erect penis.
- At ejaculation, fluid from Sertoli cells, spermatozoa and secretions from the prostate and seminal vesicles enter the prostatic region of the urethra, pass along the penile urethra and are discharged at the meatus of the urethra.

Chapter 16
The female reproductive system

In humans the female reproductive system consists of paired ovaries and the reproductive tract comprising paired uterine tubes, a uterus and a vagina (Fig. 16.1). Prior to puberty, as in males, the reproductive system in females is quiescent. At puberty, hormones from the pituitary gland initiate developmental changes which are prerequisites for reproduction. In contrast to the male reproductive system, the female system after puberty in humans is regulated by hormones secreted by the anterior pituitary gland on a monthly, cyclical basis. The cycle of activity begins at puberty and is manifested by the onset of menstruation (the loss of blood, cells and secretions from the uterus which drain through the vagina). The time when menstruation begins is known as the menarche and it occurs between 9 and 15 years of age. During each monthly menstrual cycle female oocytes differentiate and usually a single, mature oocyte is shed from an ovary each month, a process described as ovulation. The ability to produce a haploid gamete (an ovum), ovulate, conceive, support one or more developing fetuses and give birth continues from puberty until the menopause. During the menopause, which may begin between 45 and 50 years of age, the menstrual cycles and ovulation become irregular and then cease. During and beyond the menopause the hormonal signals required to stimulate the cyclical activity of the ovaries and the uterus also cease but the factor(s) that cause this cessation are not understood.

Ovaries

The ovaries are located in the pelvic cavity and are small (approximately 3 × 2 × 1.5 cm) and roughly ovoid in shape. Each ovary is attached by a stalk of double-layered membrane to the posterior surface of each side of the broad ligament (the peritoneal membrane surrounding the uterus) (Fig. 16.1).

Blood (and lymphatic) vessels and nerves pass to each ovary within this membrane. The ovary is divided into two main regions, an outer cortex and inner medulla, though the demarcation between the two is not well defined. A simple cuboidal epithelium, known as the germinal epithelium, covers the cortex of each ovary and is continuous with the peritoneal epithelium. This name arises from the erroneous supposition that 'germ' cells capable of becoming ova (the female gametes) developed from this layer. It is now known that the 'germ' cells which are the stem cells (oogonia) for female gametes develop in the embryonic yolk sac and migrate to the ovaries during fetal development in utero (see Mitchell B, Sharma R. *Embryology: An Illustrated Colour Text*. Elsevier: 2004).

Cortex of the ovary

Immediately below the germinal epithelium is a thin layer of dense irregular connective tissue, the tunica albuginea. A connective tissue stroma containing some fibroblast-like cells supports structures in the cortex known as ovarian follicles (Fig. 16.2). Ovarian follicles comprise an oogonium, or a developing oocyte, surrounded by epithelial cells. In

human females, between puberty and the menopause, ovarian follicles vary widely in appearance and size as they are in various stages of development. Some stromal cells are irregularly distributed in whorls in the cortex and others lie around developing follicles as layers known as theca (Fig. 16.2). Some of the fibroblast-like cells differentiate and are able to secrete steroid hormones.

Oogenesis and ovarian follicle development

In utero and prepubertal stages

In a developing female embryo from about the sixth week in utero, primordial, diploid oogonia migrate from the yolk sac and enter the developing ovary. From this time oogonia undergo mitosis and produce more oogonia. By about the fifth month of fetal life each ovary contains 5–7 million oogonia and migration of oogonia from the yolk sac stops. In contrast to spermatogonia, which continue to act as stem cells for spermatozoa production throughout life in males, mitosis of oogonia stops before birth and no new oogonia are formed thereafter. Indeed, the majority of oogonia die before birth.

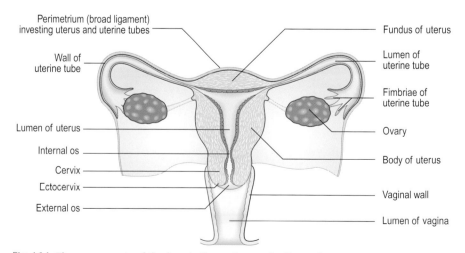

Fig. 16.1 **The components of the female (human) reproductive system.**

Perimetrium (broad ligament) investing uterus and uterine tubes

Wall of uterine tube

Lumen of uterus

Internal os

Cervix

Ectocervix

External os

Fundus of uterus

Lumen of uterine tube

Fimbriae of uterine tube

Ovary

Body of uterus

Vaginal wall

Lumen of vagina

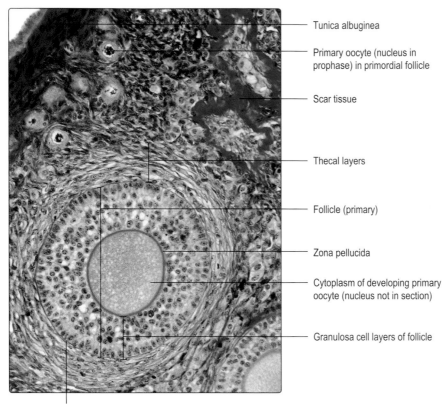

Tunica albuginea

Primary oocyte (nucleus in prophase) in primordial follicle

Scar tissue

Thecal layers

Follicle (primary)

Zona pellucida

Cytoplasm of developing primary oocyte (nucleus not in section)

Granulosa cell layers of follicle

Basement membrane of follicle

Fig. 16.2 **Ovary. A primary follicle and several small, primordial follicles are present in the cortex surrounded by connective tissue cells and fibres.** Connective tissue is stained red. Special stain. Medium magnification.

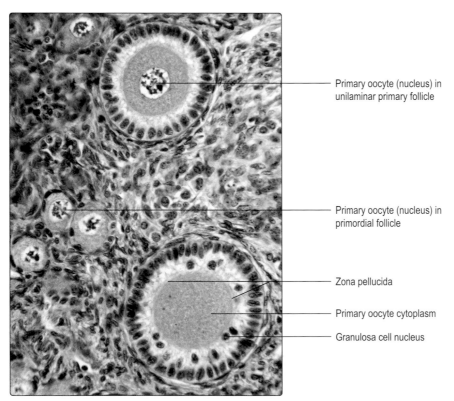

Primary oocyte (nucleus) in unilaminar primary follicle

Primary oocyte (nucleus) in primordial follicle

Zona pellucida

Primary oocyte cytoplasm

Granulosa cell nucleus

Fig. 16.3 **Ovary. Two primary and several primordial follicles.** The nucleus of the primary oocyte in one primary follicle and the nuclei in the primordial follicles have the clumped chromatin typical of cells in prophase of the first meiotic division. Special stain. High magnification.

All surviving oogonia become primary oocytes before birth as they replicate their DNA and then enter the prophase of the first (reduction) division of meiosis. This is the phase in which homologous chromosomes pair and exchange short regions of DNA, thus introducing genetic variation to the chromosomes derived originally from the mother and the father. Primary oocytes remain in the first prophase of meiosis unless they become atretic and die in the ovary or, after puberty, are shed at ovulation.

At birth there are 1–2 million primary oocytes remaining and each is surrounded by a layer of flattened epithelial cells known as follicular cells. Each primary oocyte and the surrounding follicular cells form a spherical, primordial follicle. Such follicles are predominant in the outer regions of the cortex (Fig. 16.2). Many primordial follicles die during childhood, leaving only about 400 000 at puberty.

Ovarian follicles in menstrual cycles

During each menstrual cycle several primordial follicles begin to develop but many become atretic (see below) and the oocyte dies. Usually, only one oocyte is released from a developed follicle every 28 days at ovulation, so that the lifetime total of female gametes shed is only around 400. In adults, ovarian follicles may be defined by the stage of their development and are categorised into four types: primordial, primary, secondary (antral) and Graafian (mature) follicles.

- *Primordial follicles* (Figs 16.2 and 16.3). These consist of a primary oocyte, in the prophase of the first meiotic division, surrounded by a single layer of flattened epithelial cells which is surrounded by a basement membrane.
- *Primary follicles.* Each month, several primordial follicles begin to develop and form primary follicles. This development is stimulated by follicle-stimulating hormone from the anterior pituitary gland. In each developing primary follicle the primary oocyte increases in volume and the surrounding flattened follicle cells become cuboidal or columnar in shape and are then known as granulosa cells. At this stage, the follicles are described as unilaminar primary follicles (Fig. 16.3), and they are deeper in the ovary than primordial follicles.

Unilaminar follicles become multilaminar follicles as mitotic activity is high in granulosa cells and the new cells form layers around each developing primary oocyte (Figs 16.2–16.4). During this time, the primary oocyte enlarges considerably

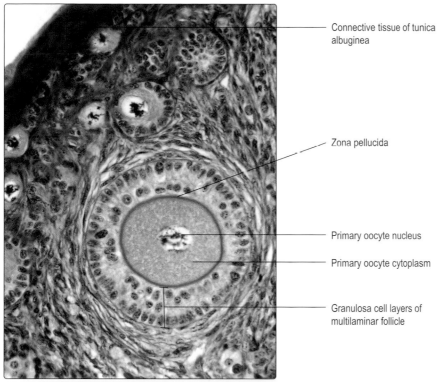

Fig. 16.4 **Ovary. Multilaminar follicle.** Connective tissue is stained red. Special stain. High magnification.

Labels (Fig. 16.4):
- Connective tissue of tunica albuginea
- Zona pellucida
- Primary oocyte nucleus
- Primary oocyte cytoplasm
- Granulosa cell layers of multilaminar follicle

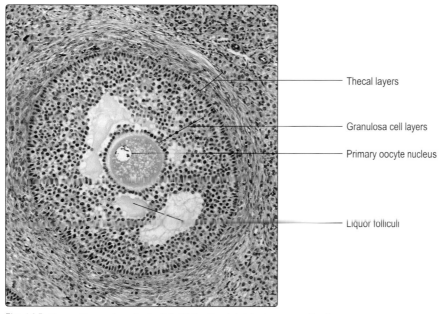

Fig. 16.5 **Ovary. Secondary (antral) follicle.** Special stain. Low magnification.

Labels (Fig. 16.5):
- Thecal layers
- Granulosa cell layers
- Primary oocyte nucleus
- Liquor folliculi

hormone from the anterior pituitary gland binds to cells of the theca interna and this stimulates them to produce steroids. These steroids are converted by granulosa cells into oestrogens (female steroid hormones). Oestrogens are involved in stimulating the uterus each month (see below) and in the development and maintenance of the secondary sexual characteristics and of the mammary glands.

- *Secondary follicles.* Some multilaminar primary follicles develop and enlarge further, under the influence of follicle-stimulating hormone. The granulosa cells produce fluid, liquor folliculi, which appears in spaces between the granulosa cells (Fig. 16.5). These follicles are described as secondary (antral) follicles. Gradually, the fluid-filled spaces coalesce into a single large space, the antrum, and development proceeds with the formation of a Graafian (mature) follicle.

- *Graafian (mature) follicles.* As the single antrum enlarges the granulosa cells appear as layers around the fluid and the layers become thinner as the follicle enlarges further. The oocyte, surrounded by granulosa cells, bulges into the fluid in the antrum and the whole bulge is known as the cumulus oophorus (Fig. 16.6).

  Graafian follicles may become very large (2.5 cm in diameter) and bulge from the surface of the ovary prior to ovulation. The primary oocyte (which was arrested in utero in prophase of the first reduction meiotic division) completes the first meiotic division just prior to ovulation. The result is one large secondary oocyte with half the original number of chromosomes (23 in humans) and a small cell, known as the first polar body (also with 23 chromosomes), which degenerates.

Atresia of follicles

Most developing follicles fail to become mature Graafian follicles. Atresia may occur at any stage of follicle development and it involves the death of granulosa cells (Fig. 16.7) and the oocyte. Atretic follicles are gradually replaced by scar tissue containing fibroblasts and collagen (Fig. 16.2).

and a prominent deposit of condensed material known as the zona pellucida appears between the oocyte and the granulosa cells (Figs 16.2–16.4). Primary oocytes, which may grow to 120 μm in diameter, may appear to lack a nucleus (Figs 16.2 and 16.3) in routine histological sections which, at only 5–10 μm thick, can fail to include the nucleus. As primary follicles grow the basement membrane which

separates the (epithelial) granulosa cells from surrounding connective tissue (Fig. 16.2) becomes more apparent.

Stromal cells around each primary follicle form two layers during this phase: the theca interna and theca externa. The inner theca is well vascularised whereas the outer theca is composed of fibrous connective tissue, although the layers are not always distinct (Fig. 16.2). Luteinising

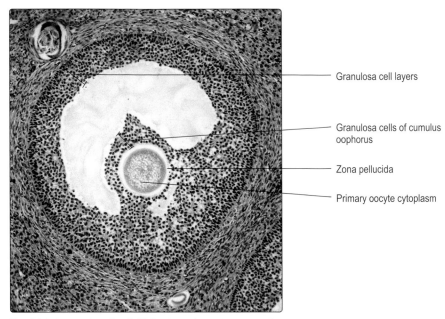

Fig. 16.6 **Ovary, Graafian follicle.** Special stain. Low magnification.

- Granulosa cell layers
- Granulosa cells of cumulus oophorus
- Zona pellucida
- Primary oocyte cytoplasm

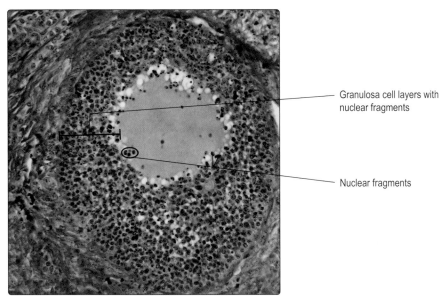

- Granulosa cell layers with nuclear fragments
- Nuclear fragments

Fig. 16.7 **Ovary. Atretic follicle.** Densely stained fragments of DNA and disruption of the layers of granulosa cells characterise atretic follicles. This follicle is large and had developed into a secondary follicle. The developing primary oocyte is not in the plane of section but it too will be undergoing degeneration. Connective tissue is stained red. Special stain. Low magnification.

Ovulation

Ovulation usually happens once at the mid-point (day 14) of every menstrual cycle. It is the process whereby a secondary oocyte and the surrounding cluster of granulosa cells (the corona radiata) are expelled from a Graafian follicle and away from the surface of the ovary. Ovulation is brought about as the increasing volume of the Graafian follicle puts pressure onto the tunica albuginea and surface epithelium of the ovary and also compresses blood vessels in the region. This is coincidental with a breakdown of the wall of the follicle in the same region. The oocyte, granulosa cells forming the corona radiata and fluid burst from the antrum of the follicle and enter the peritoneal cavity. Further development of the oocyte normally occurs only if it passes from the peritoneal cavity into the lumen of the uterine tube (see below).

Formation of a corpus luteum

After ovulation, under the influence of luteinising hormone from the anterior pituitary gland, a corpus luteum develops. It forms from the remnants of granulosa cells from the ruptured Graafian follicle, and cells and blood vessels which grow into these remnants from the theca interna. The theca and granulosa cells forming the corpus luteum begin to secrete female steroid hormones, mainly progesterone. The secretory cells pack the corpus luteum (Fig. 16.8), which may grow into a sphere up to about 2 cm in diameter by day 25 of the menstrual cycle. The progesterone secreted by the corpus luteum is essential in preparing the uterus for the possible arrival of a fertilised ovum and the establishment of pregnancy.

If pregnancy is established the corpus luteum doubles in size and is an essential source of progesterone during the first months of pregnancy in humans. If fertilisation and implantation do not occur, the corpus luteum degenerates, a scar forms from fibroblasts and collagen fibres, and the resultant structure, known as a corpus albicans, persists in the ovary for some time.

Medulla of the ovary

The medulla is the central core of the ovary and it is surrounded by the cortex except where vessels and nerves are connected to the ovary. Stromal cells, similar to those in the cortex, are present in the medulla but follicles are not present.

Uterine tube and fertilisation

Uterine tubes

Each uterine tube in humans is about 10 cm long. The lumen at one end of each tube is open to the peritoneal cavity. This end is formed by frilly, finger-like projections (fimbriae) of the tube. Fimbriae are important in helping guide the oocyte (released at ovulation into the peritoneal cavity) into the lumen of the uterine tube. The other end of the uterine tube opens into the uterus (Fig.

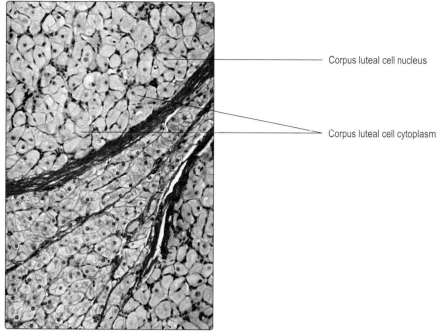

Fig. 16.8 **Ovary. Corpus luteum.** Connective tissue is stained red. Special stain. Medium magnification.

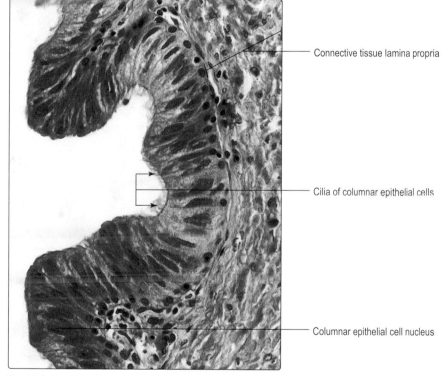

Fig. 16.9 **Uterine tube.** High magnification.

16.1). The structure of each uterine tube consists of three layers:

- *The inner layer is a mucosa.* The mucosa is highly folded and consists of simple columnar epithelial cells on a basement membrane and a thin, supporting connective tissue lamina propria (Fig. 16.9). Some epithelial cells have cilia and others do not. The non-ciliated cells are secretory and the fluid they produce provides an environment in the lumen of the tube in which the (secondary) oocyte and spermatozoa can survive and fertilisation can occur. The ciliated cells beat and assist in wafting the oocyte toward the uterus. The fluid flow towards the uterus must not be stronger than the ability of spermatozoa to swim from the uterus and along the tube. The fluid in the uterine tube and its direction of flow towards the uterus also help to prevent the passage of microorganisms into and along the uterine tubes and into the peritoneal cavity.

- *The middle layer is a muscularis.* There are two, thin, ill-defined layers of smooth muscle cells, an inner circular and an outer longitudinal layer. Peristaltic contractions of the smooth muscle cells assist in moving the contents of the lumen.

- *The outer layer is a thin covering of serosa.* This layer is continuous with the broad ligament covering the uterus.

Fertilisation

Once a secondary oocyte, surrounded by cells of the cumulus oophorus, enters the uterine tube it remains there for 2–3 days, during which time it is capable of being fertilised by a spermatozoon. At this stage, it has started the second (mitotic) division of meiosis but is suspended in metaphase pending possible fertilisation by a spermatozoon.

Fertilisation occurs in the uterine tube when a spermatozoon passes between cells of the cumulus oophorus and penetrates the cytoplasmic membrane of the oocyte. Once fertilised, the oocyte completes meiosis and this restores the diploid number of chromosomes. (A second polar body is released at this division and degenerates.) The fertilised oocyte undergoes rapid rounds of cell division (mitosis) and develops into a blastocyst. Further details of the subsequent development of the blastocyst are described elsewhere (see Mitchell B, Sharma R. *Embryology: An Illustrated Colour Text.* Elsevier: 2004).

After fertilisation, the blastocyst passes to the uterus, carried there in the fluid flowing from the uterine tube. The timing of the arrival of the blastocyst in the uterus is critical. The blastocyst has to be sufficiently developed so that it is able to attach to the uterine epithelium. In addition, it must arrive in the uterus when, and not before, the uterus is in a receptive state. This state is dependent on progesterone from the corpus luteum (see below).

Uterus

The uterus in humans is a single midline organ. It is able to accommodate and facilitate the development of the blastocyst and differentiation of the embryo and its further growth as a fetus. In addition, the uterus supports the development of the placenta and expels the fetus and placenta at parturition. The uterus is divided into three regions (Fig. 16.1). The superior part is the fundus. The body is the largest part of the uterus, into which the uterine tubes open. The most inferior part of the uterus is the cervix, which projects and opens into the vagina.

The wall of the uterus in the fundus and body regions is composed of three layers: endometrium, myometrium and perimetrium.

■ *Endometrium*. This is a mucosa; it forms the inner layer and varies in structure under the influence of oestrogens and progesterone (see below). The endometrium has an inner basal layer and a superficial (functional) layer. A simple, columnar epithelium lines the uterine lumen and branched tubular glands dip deep into the connective tissue of the lamina propria and extend to the myometrium (Fig. 16.10). Some of the epithelial cells are secretory and others have cilia.

The superficial layer of the endometrium is shed at menstruation or, if pregnancy occurs, adapts and functions as a support for the blastocyst and the developing placenta and embryo (and its development into a fetus). Within the superficial layer there are helical arteries. These supply the endometrium as it increases in thickness in response to the hormonal changes occurring during the menstrual cycle (and in pregnancy). It is from the capillaries supplied by these vessels that blood is lost during menstruation. The inner basal layer of the endometrium is a relatively narrow region, though highly significant, since it is this layer that undergoes cellular proliferation and replaces the superficial layer shed at menstruation.

■ *Myometrium*. This is the muscularis of the uterus. It is composed of three or four thick and ill-defined layers of smooth muscle. Arcuate arteries in the middle of the myometrium supply the helical arteries in the endometrium. Hypertrophy and hyperplasia of smooth muscle cells are stimulated by oestrogen and these changes are particularly important in pregnancy. Contractions of the myometrium are stimulated by oxytocin from the posterior pituitary (Chapter 14) and by prostaglandins from the region of the uterus in pregnancy known as decidua (see Mitchell B, Sharma R. *Embryology: An Illustrated Colour Text*. Elsevier: 2004). These contractions result in expulsion of the fetus and placenta at parturition.

■ *Perimetrium* (Fig. 16.1). The thin, outer, serosal (peritoneal) covering of the uterus is known as the perimetrium. It consists of a single layer of squamous epithelial cells beneath which is loose connective tissue attached to the myometrium. The perimetrium invests most of the uterus as the broad ligament, encloses vessels and nerves passing to the uterus and is continuous with the peritoneum. As the uterus expands during pregnancy the fluid secreted onto the surface of the perimetrium by its epithelial cells ensures relatively friction-free movement between the uterus and adjacent structures such as gut tubes.

Cervix of the uterus

The cervix is the lower part of the uterus, and the lower part of the cervix projects into the vagina as the ectocervix (Fig. 16.1). In the cervix, the smooth muscle forming the myometrial layer in the rest of the uterus is mostly replaced by connective tissue containing collagen and elastin fibres. The lumen of the cervix communicates with the lumen of the body of the uterus at the internal os and opens into the vagina at the external os.

The lumen of the cervix is lined by a simple columnar epithelium. Deep slits and tubes, lined by columnar epithelial cells, extend into the connective tissue of the cervical wall. Cervical epithelial cells are palely stained in routine (H&E)

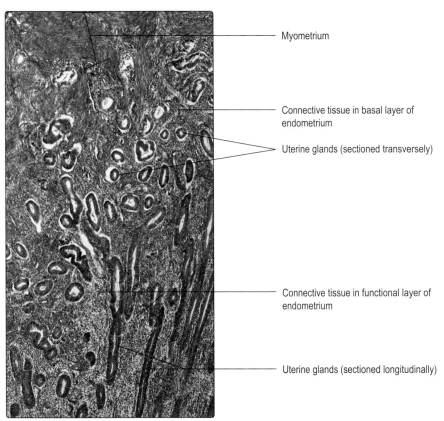

Myometrium

Connective tissue in basal layer of endometrium

Uterine glands (sectioned transversely)

Connective tissue in functional layer of endometrium

Uterine glands (sectioned longitudinally)

Fig. 16.10 **Uterus. Body region, proliferative phase.** Very low magnification.

Clinical note

Ectopic pregnancy Sometimes a developing blastocyst becomes arrested in its passage from the uterine tube to the uterus. It may then develop and attach to the mucosal epithelium of the uterine tube. The wall of the uterine tube is not able to sustain the developing blastocyst for long and blood vessels in the wall of the tube rupture. The result is haemorrhage, possibly into the peritoneal cavity and possibly into the uterus and showing as a vaginal discharge. These events usually cause severe pain and loss of the embryo and can cause death of the woman.

histological preparations (Fig. 16.11) in contrast to the rest of the uterus. Cervical epithelial cells synthesise and secrete mucus, which is rich in carbohydrates. This mucus does not stain strongly in routine preparations. Cervical mucus varies in viscosity during the menstrual cycle. The mucus is relatively watery at mid-cycle when ovulation occurs, but more viscous at other times and during pregnancy. The thicker mucus helps prevent the entry of microorganisms into the uterus. The watery mucus provides relatively little resistance to swimming spermatozoa during the short time after ovulation that an oocyte is available for fertilisation in the uterine tube. Cervical mucus drains to the vagina and acts as a lubricant during sexual intercourse. The surface of the cervix where it projects into the vagina is covered by stratified, squamous, non-keratinising epithelium, similar to that which lines the vagina itself (see below).

The menstrual cycle

The menstrual cycle occurring in human females mainly affects the reproductive system, particularly the ovaries and the uterus. The cycle lasts for an average of 28 days and is described as having three phases: menstrual, proliferative (follicular) and secretory (luteal).

- *Menstrual phase.* Conventionally, the menstrual cycle is said to begin as blood is lost from the vagina at the start of menstruation. The phase lasts until vaginal bleeding stops (after about 4 days). Menstruation occurs, if fertilisation has not occurred, as a result of a rapid fall in the levels of progesterone (and oestrogen) secreted by cells in the corpus luteum in the last 2 or 3 days of the cycle. At the start of the menstrual phase the endometrium is thick and the glands are distended and have a characteristic shape (Fig. 16.12). The superficial (functional) layer is shed during this phase and bleeding occurs from damaged vessels in the endometrium. At the end of this phase only the basal layer remains intact.
- *Proliferative (follicular) phase.* After menstruation, the damaged endometrium is repaired as epithelial, stromal and endothelial cells in the basal layer proliferate and replace the shed functional layer with straight tubular glands and

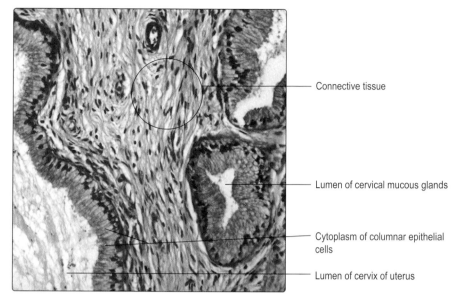

Fig. 16.11 **Cervix of uterus.** Medium magnification.

Connective tissue

Lumen of cervical mucous glands

Cytoplasm of columnar epithelial cells

Lumen of cervix of uterus

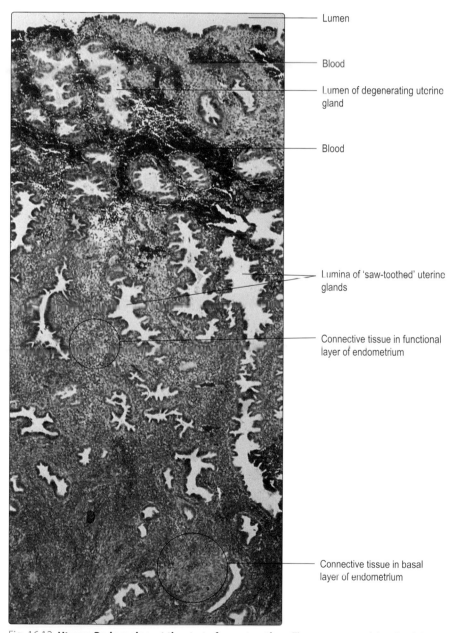

Lumen

Blood

Lumen of degenerating uterine gland

Blood

Lumina of 'saw-toothed' uterine glands

Connective tissue in functional layer of endometrium

Connective tissue in basal layer of endometrium

Fig. 16.12 **Uterus. Body region, at the start of menstruation.** The appearance of the glands is typical of the secretory stage. The distribution of blood shows that menstruation has started. Very low magnification.

connective tissue stroma (Fig. 16.10). This phase lasts from about day 5 of the cycle to about day 14. The proliferative and repair activities are regulated indirectly by follicle-stimulating hormone (FSH) from the anterior pituitary gland. FSH stimulates the growth of ovarian follicles and as the number of granulosa cells increases they secrete increasing levels of oestrogen into the blood. The timing of the secretion of these oestrogens and the effect they have on endometrial repair is important because it helps to ensure that the uterus is in a receptive state appropriate for the arrival of a blastocyst.

- *Secretory (luteal) phase.* This phase begins after ovulation (on day 14) and lasts until menstruation (i.e. from day 15 to day 28). After ovulation, luteinising hormone (LH) from the anterior pituitary stimulates the formation of the corpus luteum, which secretes progesterone. In this phase, under the influence of progesterone, the whole endometrium becomes thicker and oedematous and the glands deepen and become saw-toothed in shape (Fig. 16.12). The epithelial cells accumulate glycogen and secrete glycoproteins into the lumen, activities which could provide nourishment for a developing blastocyst. The timing of these events is also essential in preparing the endometrium for the blastocyst, particularly as the uterine secretions will nourish the developing embryo prior to the formation of the placenta.

The vagina

The vagina is a fibromuscular tube that leads from the uterus to the exterior. The wall of the vagina consists of three layers: an inner mucosa, a fibromuscular layer and an outer connective tissue covering which attaches the vagina to adjacent structures, e.g. the urethra.

The vaginal mucosa, in humans, comprises a non-keratinising, stratified, squamous epithelium and a connective tissue lamina propria. Cells in the upper layers of the vaginal epithelium are characterised by their content of glycogen, which is extracted during routine histological processing and so the cells appear empty (Fig. 16.13). The surface epithelial cells are gradually shed and replaced by

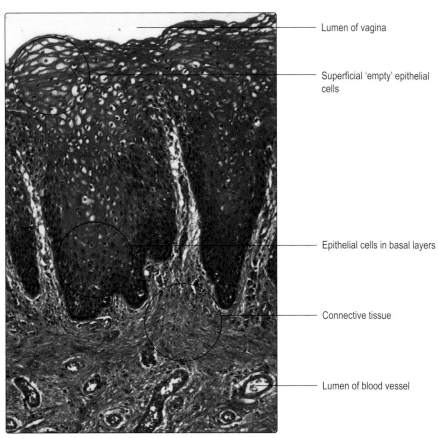

Lumen of vagina

Superficial 'empty' epithelial cells

Epithelial cells in basal layers

Connective tissue

Lumen of blood vessel

Fig. 16.13 **Vagina.** Low magnification.

cells arising from stem cells in the basal layer. Glycogen, released from shed cells, is metabolised by non-pathogenic bacteria in the vaginal lumen and lactic acid is released. This symbiosis is important as the lactic acid maintains a low pH in the vaginal lumen and this provides a hostile environment for many types of pathogenic bacteria which could gain access to the upper parts of the tract (and the peritoneal cavity). The wall of the vagina mostly comprises fibrous connective tissue, which includes mainly collagen and elastin fibres. Some smooth muscle cells are also present. During sexual stimulation, cervical mucus and a watery transudate from the vaginal wall facilitate the entry of the penis during sexual intercourse.

Mammary glands

Mammary glands are paired structures lying on the anterior chest wall. After puberty in human females the glands develop under the influence of oestrogen and progesterone (mainly from the ovaries). During pregnancy and lactation oestrogen, progesterone and prolactin (from the anterior pituitary gland) further stimulate the glands. In females, mammary glands secrete milk, the defining substance for nourishing the offspring of mammals. Mammary glands are also present in males, though considerably less well developed. It is important to recognise their presence in males since, like their counterparts in females, they too may develop cancer.

Mammary glands are classified as compound tubuloalveolar glands (Chapter 3). Each gland contains about 20 lobes separated by connective tissue, and each lobe drains through a lactiferous duct to a nipple. Connective tissue comprising collagen, fibroblasts and adipose cells separates each lobe and supports the tubuloalveolar glands within the lobes. The number of adipose cells present varies from individual to individual.

Mammary glands in non-pregnant women are in a resting state. Within each lobe there are lobules comprising clusters of epithelial-lined ducts (Fig. 16.14) separated by loose connective tissue, but there are no secretory cells. During pregnancy, under the influence of hormones (oestrogen, progesterone and prolactin) the epithelial cells of the ducts proliferate, the duct system extends, and spherical clusters of secretory cells form as alveoli at the ends of the ducts. Ducts and alveoli swell and fill the lobules. The secretory alveoli are lined by cuboidal epithelial cells and are surrounded by myoepithelial cells. The epithelial cells synthesise and secrete milk, which is released from the nipple post partum. During lactation, alveoli may appear distended with secretion (Fig. 16.15). The expulsion of milk is stimulated by suckling. It involves the secretion of oxytocin (from the posterior pituitary) and the contraction of myoepithelial cells surrounding the alveolar epithelium.

Milk contains proteins, lipids, lactose (milk sugar), minerals and vitamins, which together constitute the nutrition required by infants. Milk also contains antibodies and various immune cells. At this early stage, the infant has little immunity of its own and the passage of antibodies in milk from the mother is the principal means by which a newborn is afforded some immune protection from potential microbiological invaders from their new world.

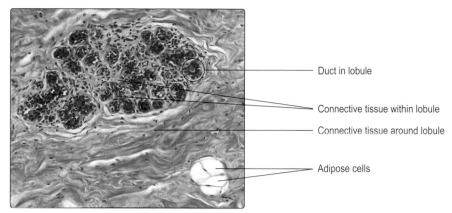

Fig. 16.14 **Breast in non-pregnant, non-lactating female.** Medium magnification.

- Duct in lobule
- Connective tissue within lobule
- Connective tissue around lobule
- Adipose cells

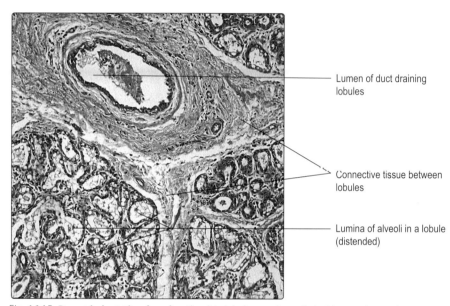

Fig. 16.15 **Breast in lactating female.** Alveoli in lobules are distended with secretion and are apparent at this low magnification. It is possible to identify only a large duct in interlobular connective tissue but not ducts in the lobules. Low magnification.

- Lumen of duct draining lobules
- Connective tissue between lobules
- Lumina of alveoli in a lobule (distended)

> ### Clinical note
>
> **Breast cancer** The most common swellings and disorders occurring in breasts are not cancerous. However, the epithelial cells lining the ducts in the breast may become cancerous in women (and men) and produce lumps or distortions. Spread of cancerous cells from the breast occurs via the rich network of blood and lymphatic vessels in the breast. Early diagnosis of the cell types present in breast lumps and appropriate treatment improves survival rates.

Summary

The female reproductive system

- This consists of paired ovaries and the reproductive tract (paired uterine tubes, a single uterus (in humans) and a vagina).

Ovaries

- Ovaries contain ovarian follicles, which contain oocytes.
- Each month, after puberty, several follicles begin to grow:
  - follicle cells increase in number and are known as granulosa cells; they surround a developing oocyte and secrete mainly oestrogens.
- Usually, only one follicle grows to maturity each month and one oocyte is shed at ovulation (other developing follicles become atretic and die).
- After ovulation, a corpus luteum develops from the remnants of the follicle and a surrounding layer (theca) of connective tissue cells and blood vessels.
- The pituitary hormones follicle-stimulating hormone and luteinising hormone, respectively, control the development of follicles and corpora lutea.
- If fertilisation does not occur the corpus luteum degenerates, progesterone levels fall and menstruation occurs.
- If fertilisation occurs, the corpus luteum grows and secretes progesterone, which prepares the uterus to support the developing embryo until the placenta forms.

Uterine tubes

- These are lined by a simple epithelium composed of secretory and ciliated cells.
- They have sparse connective tissue lamina propria connecting the epithelium to a muscularis of two layers of smooth muscle.
- They are covered by a serosal (peritoneal) membrane.
- They receive the oocyte after ovulation, are the site of fertilisation and transfer the blastocyst to the uterus.

Uterus

- A simple epithelium lines most of the uterus and glands dip into the mucosa as far as the muscularis externa:
  - most of the mucosa is shed at menstruation and bleeding occurs
  - after menstruation, the remaining cells in the basal mucosal layer proliferate (under the influence of oestrogens) and repair the superficial layer
  - after ovulation (under the influence of progesterone) the mucosa thickens, the epithelial cells begin to store glycogen and secrete glycoproteins. The glands become saw-toothed in shape.
- The muscularis externae is formed of several layers of smooth muscle which undergoes hyperplasia and hypertrophy during pregnancy.
- Part of the uterus, the cervix, is lined by columnar epithelial cells which secrete mucus. The outer wall of the cervix is formed mostly of connective tissue.

Vagina

- A stratified squamous epithelium lines the vagina and the upper cells contain glycogen.
- The vaginal wall is formed largely by connective tissue.

Glossary

Acinus a spherical unit of secretory cells in an exocrine gland.

Adenoma an abnormal growth of glandular epithelial cells that is non-cancerous.

Adluminal refers to structures adjacent to the lumen of a tube.

Allergen a substance capable of provoking an immune (allergic) reaction in an individual involving the production of specific immunoglobulins.

Alveolus a small cavity, e.g. the blind-ended epithelial sacs at the ends of airways in the lungs.

Anaphylaxis an excessive (sometimes fatal) specific reaction to allergens that results from breakdown of mast cell granules and leads to sudden hypotension and severe bronchoconstriction.

Anastomosis a union or joining together of parts, e.g. of arteries, often forming a network.

Antibody a protein (immunoglobulin) produced as part of an immune response to a specific molecule (antigen) and able to bind specifically with that molecule.

Antigen a molecule (protein or carbohydrate) capable of stimulating the production of an antibody.

Apoptosis programmed cell death (programmed in the DNA).

Benign non-cancerous (harmless).

Blastocyst the stage reached when the solid mass of cells which have developed from a fertilised egg form a hollow structure comprising two distinct components. One component will form the placenta and the other an embryo.

Bronchoscopy a technique in which a flexible telescope is introduced into a patient's trachea to inspect the interior of the bronchi.

Cancer a general term applied to any malignant growth (tumour) with potentially unlimited growth and spread; it is usually fatal if untreated.

Cancerous refers to cancer.

Carcinoma a malignant tumour formed by an abnormal growth of epithelial cells that penetrate their basement membrane and spread to other sites.

Cell the basic unit of living organisms.

Chromosome a linear structure in the nucleus that contains hereditary material (DNA and associated proteins) in the form of genes.

Cilium a projection from the apical (opposite to the basal) surface of a cell containing a core of microtubules capable of moving the cilium. In the respiratory tract, coordinated beating of many cilia on individual cells moves particles out of the tract.

Circadian cyclical activity occurring over a 24 hour period.

Diploid the number of chromosomes in somatic cells of a species comprising pairs of homologous chromosomes and a pair of sex chromosomes. This is twice the number present in the germ cells (ova and spermatozoa). (There are 22 pairs of homologous chromosomes and a pair of sex chromosomes in humans.)

Effete worn out or dying.

Extracellular outside the cell.

Fusiform a long structure narrowing at each end like a spindle.

Gamete a mature male or female germ cell which contains the haploid number of chromosomes. A male gamete (spermatozoon) fertilises a female gamete (oocyte), and forms a zygote (with the diploid number of chromosomes) which develops into a new individual.

Genitalia external reproductive structures of each sex.

Germ cells primitive, undifferentiated reproductive cells (oogonia in females and spermatozoa in males).

Haemorrhage escape of blood from vessels.

Haploid the set of chromosomes found in germ cells (i.e. the 23 chromosomes in human germ cells).

Hilum a depressed region on the surface of some organs, e.g. the kidney, where structures enter or leave the organ.

Histochemistry the application of chemical reactions to sections of tissues to demonstrate certain chemical components.

Histopathologist a specialist in diagnosing abnormalities by examining tissue sections using a microscope.

Homeostasis the physiological changes which occur and ensure relatively constant conditions are maintained within the body of living organisms.

Homologous similar.

Humoral blood borne.

Hypertonic indicates a fluid with a higher concentration of solutes than in blood plasma.

Hypotonic indicates a fluid with a lower concentration of solutes than in blood plasma.

Immunohistochemistry the application of labelled antibodies to demonstrate specific antigens in tissue sections.

Inflammation (inflammatory reaction) dilation of blood capillaries, increased vascular permeability and infiltration of immune cells, including neutrophils, macrophages, lymphocytes and plasma cells to the site. Redness, swelling, tenderness and pain may occur.

Interstitium region lying between cells, often occupied by tissue fluid.

Intracellular within a cell.

Isotonic indicates a fluid with the same concentration of solutes as blood plasma.

In vitro literally in glass. Not in living individuals, e.g. in tissue culture systems.

Lumen hollow centre of a tubular structure or organ, e.g. urinary bladder.

Malignant harmful or cancerous, applied to the uncontrolled proliferation and growth of cancer cells.

Matrix extracellular matrix is the material outside cells, and intracellular matrix the components of the cytoplasm within cells supporting the organelles and cytoskeleton.

Meatus an opening to the outside of the body.

Mesenchyme primitive embryonic connective tissue.

Mesentery the double-layered serosal (peritoneal) membrane attaching many regions of the gut to the posterior abdominal wall and supporting vessels passing to and from the gut.

Metastasis the process whereby malignant, cancerous cells spread to distant sites from their original site (i.e. the primary tumour). Also a mass of cancerous cells growing at a (secondary) site distant from their original site.

Microorganism life forms visible only with a microscope, e.g. bacteria and viruses.

Mucous membrane an epithelium (and its supporting connective tissue) that covers inner surfaces of the body (a mucosa). Most mucous membranes secrete mucus which keeps the surface moist.

Mucus a secretion of complexes of large carbohydrate molecules and proteins which are viscous (slimy).

Neoplasm a new growth which may originate from any of the primary tissues and may be benign or malignant.

Neuroendocrine indicates cells derived from the neural crest in the embryo, dispersed in the body which secrete hormones. Some secretions have both local and systemic effects; some act as neurotransmitters.

Oedema swelling in tissues caused by excessive accumulation of tissue fluid.

Organ a collection of primary tissues joined in a specific location and carrying out specific functions.

Organelle a specific structure in cell cytoplasm with a particular function.

Organism a fundamental life form capable of independent existence.

Papilla a projection from a surface of a tissue or organ. It may have a specific normal purpose or be abnormal.

Paracrine indicates a type of secretion exerting local effects, e.g. as carried out by some neuroendocrine cells.

Parenchyma the main cell type in an organ associated with its principal function.

Parietal related to the wall of a cavity.

Pelvic cavity the lower part of the trunk containing pelvic organs.

Peritoneum the serous membrane investing the walls of the abdominopelvic cavity and covering the organs contained therein.

Pheromone a naturally occurring molecule from an individual that evokes a behavioural response via the olfactory system of an individual of the same species.

Photomicrograph a photograph taken using a microscope and camera.

Prostaglandins a class of molecule derived from fatty acids that are widely produced in the body and act locally on a variety of cells, e.g. they affect the contraction of the smooth muscle in the uterus in pregnancy and affect blood flow in many regions.

Serous membrane membrane that lines the walls of, and covers organs in, the three cavities of the trunk, i.e. the pericardial, pleural and abdominal cavities.

Somatic of the body. Describes all the cells of the body except the male and female germ cells. The somatic nervous system is that part of the system under conscious control.

Stroma the connective tissue supporting parenchyma.

Synovial one of the three different types of joint, characterised by a synovial membrane lining the capsule of the joint (and by articulating surfaces covered by hyaline cartilage).

System (of the body) a group of organs and structures carrying out specific, related functions.

Tissue the material from which the body is made: there are four primary tissue types (epithelial, connective, muscle and nerve).

Tract anatomically connected and functionally related structures, e.g. gastrointestinal tract. Also refers to a bundle of nerve cell cytoplasmic processes passing through the brain or spinal cord.

Tumour a mass of cells (usually abnormal) which proliferate and grow abnormally.

Vasoactive amine an amine that influences the calibre of blood vessels.

Visceral of an organ (especially in the thorax or abdomen).

Index

Figures and tables are comprehensively referred to from the text. Therefore, significant material in figures and tables have only been given a page reference in the absence of their concomitant mention in the text referring to that figure. Entries in bold indicate references to the glossary.